SOMEBODY I USED
TO KNOW

SOMEBODY I USED TO KNOW

WENDY MITCHELL

with Anna Wharton

BLOOMSBURY

LONDON · OXFORD · NEW YORK · NEW DELHI · SYDNEY

Bloomsbury Publishing
An imprint of Bloomsbury Publishing Plc

50 Bedford Square   1385 Broadway
London   New York
WC1B 3DP   NY 10018
UK   USA

www.bloomsbury.com

BLOOMSBURY and the Diana logo are trademarks of Bloomsbury Publishing Plc

British Library Cataloguing-in-Publication Data
A catalogue record for this book is available from the British Library.

ISBN: HB: 978-1-4088-9336-4
         TPB: 978-1-4088-9337-1
       EPUB: 978-1-4088-9334-0

2 4 6 8 10 9 7 5 3 1

Typeset by Integra Software Services Pvt. Ltd.
Printed and bound in Great Britain by CPI Group (UK) Ltd, Croydon CR0 4YY

To find out more about our authors and books visit www.bloomsbury.com.
Here you will find extracts, author interviews, details of forthcoming
events and the option to sign up for our newsletters.

It happened again the other day. This was nothing like before. It was much, much worse. It wasn't a word lost from the tip of my tongue; it wasn't an absent adjective, a vanished verb. It wasn't getting up from the sofa and padding into the kitchen in slippers, then forgetting to bring back the cup of tea I'd just poured myself. It wasn't running upstairs for something and then reaching the top step and not for the life of me remembering what it might be.

This was totally different.

This was totally blank.

A

> *big*

>> *dark*

>>> *black*

>>>> *hole.*

And the worse thing was, just when I needed you most, you were gone.

***

I am running along the path by the river with an impending sense of something I can't put my finger on. It has lingered for a few weeks now. More honestly, a few months. How can I describe it? Perhaps that in itself is why I haven't been to the doctor's, why I haven't mentioned it to anyone else, not even my daughters. How are you meant to describe these things? My head feels fuzzy, life is a little less sharp. What use would that generic description be? It would be better not to waste my GP's time, and yet I know there's something, an inkling that I am function-ing around average. Even though I know that what I consider to be average would be above average for most people, this just isn't me.

It was this fuzziness that had pulled me from the sofa this afternoon, that pushed my feet into my running shoes, that placed my house keys into one hand, my iPod into another. I wasn't sure where I'd get the energy to run, but I knew I'd find it: I'd push through that initial wall, just as I had dozens of times before, and the next time I open the front door of my riverside apartment it would be with adrenalin pumping through my veins; I'd feel invigorated. That's what a run had always done.

I glance down at my feet doing their job, finding the pace the way they always did, the rhythm, the gentle thud as I hit the concrete, and I look up again at the path, waiting for the world to sharpen into focus just as it always had. 'Five hundred metres,' the robotic voice in my headphones announces, my iPod synced up to my shoes, motivation to push me through, and yet right now, it feels more like a marker of failure. I've done more than this. I tackled the Three Peaks Challenge last year and I can still conjure up the feeling I had when I reached the top of the first peak, Pen-y-ghent, more than 2,000 feet above sea level; it felt like I'd conquered the world. The same adrenalin I now desperately awaited had pushed blood around my body to tackle two more peaks on the same day, the wind blowing hard in my ears at the top. Life wasn't fuzzy around the edges then; it was pin-sharp.

It's cold and crisp and my running leggings hug my thighs, keeping the warmth of my body trapped inside. Aside from the sound of my rubber soles hitting the path, the only other sound is the swish of oars breaking the stillness of the river as the scullers practise their skills between bridges. Down one side of the river I'll go, crossing the Millennium Bridge, back up the other side, a route I have trodden so many times before. But then, in a second, everything changes. Without warning, I'm falling. There's no time to even put my hands out towards the concrete as it comes crashing towards me. My face hits the ground first; white pain shoots through my nose, my cheekbones; I feel a crack. Something hot and sticky bursts from within. It's a couple of seconds before there is complete stillness. I use it to catch my breath and when I reach up to my face my hand returns to me covered in blood. That's when the pain hits, not just physical pain, but the sting of humiliation as I look down at my legs, a tangle in front of me, and for that split second I don't recognise them or what they've done to me. Or, rather, what they've allowed to happen. I've broken my nose, I'm sure of it. I stagger to my feet, blood soaking my running top, seeping into each thread of the fabric. Helpless to stop the stain spreading further across my chest, I stumble back towards home.

My doctor's surgery is just around the corner, and so I decide to walk there and see the nurse. The shock is settling into my bones now, and by the time I stand in front of her, my hands are shaking. My knees are doing the same, and I'm hoping that she hasn't noticed.

She sends me straight to A & E and on the walk there, I'm still trying to work out what went wrong, whether it was anything to do with that sense of something I couldn't put my finger on when I set off. Was that it? Was that what I was waiting for? A fall while I was running? But somehow it feels bigger than that. I wait in A & E, the blood drying brown on my running top, tissues speckled scarlet scrunched tight inside my palm, telling myself that this is a one-off, and then finally I'm called in to see the nurse who will patch me up.

'Well, there's nothing broken,' she says. 'You're lucky. How did it happen?'

'I'm not sure,' I say. 'I was out running.'

'Ah, the perils of running,' she laughs. 'I know them well!'

We share the joke, rolling our eyes, but it's there again, that sense of something more. I'm already planning to go back along the route on my way home, to find the wonky paving slab that has left me with two black eyes, yet thankfully, no broken bones. I'm grateful that I'm on annual leave, that I don't need to walk into the office tomorrow with black and purple patterns stretched across my face.

An hour later I'm standing in front of the place where I fell. It's easily recognisable from the spatter of red where my face hit the pavement. I search all around, but there is no dip in the pavement, no loose slab, nothing to trip over. So what was it, then? The fog in my head makes it hard to decipher – there's nothing, no clues – but this has never happened before. I return home and lie back into the sofa cushions, battered and bruised, back where I was before, looking out at the River Ouse as the sky darkens above it and the mystery deepens beneath. I'm tired now, more tired than before. It hurts to close my eyes, but this time I let the lethargy cover me like a blanket, and for the first time, I don't attempt to fight it.

***

It's a few days later, and I book an appointment with my GP, the tiredness dragging me there rather than anything else. My lack of energy: that's how it started.

I sit in front of him. 'I just … I just feel slower than usual,' I say, and he studies me for a second or two.

I've been entertaining silly thoughts. One that passed through quickly was a brain tumour. I study the doctor's face to see if he's thinking the same, but he gives away no clues. Instead, his shoulders slump away from his ears and he attempts an expression of something like empathy.

'You're fit, you exercise, you eat well, you don't smoke and at fifty-six, you're relatively young,' he says. 'But there comes a time when we all have to admit to ourselves that we're just slowing down.'

He sits back in his chair then and folds his arms, waiting for it to sink in.

'You work hard, Wendy,' he sighs. 'Maybe take some time off.'

I want to tell him that I have done, that right now I'm in the middle of annual leave and the idea of taking any more than that is preposterous to someone like me. I'm the person at work who knows the system for rostering nursing shifts inside out. I'm the one my colleagues nickname 'the guru' because my recall is so sharp, because I can problem-solve in a second, reminding anyone who asks who works night shifts, who needs which day off. They can't possibly manage without me. But he's tidying papers on his desk and I sense this is the end of the appointment.

'Age,' he shrugs when he turns back and finds me staring at him.

I leave his office. I know I should be feeling relieved. My doctor isn't worried, it seems, and normally I would distract myself with work, throwing myself back into the job I love, yet I go home to an empty flat. I don't tell my daughters Gemma or Sarah about the fall. I tell myself the doctor is right, that it is nothing but age, but more months go by and the snowdrift that seems to have settled in my mind remains, along with the lack of energy and the same feeling I just can't put my finger on. There are other things too; a forgetfulness. I go on other runs and I always get to the same spot, the place where I fell, and check the pavement every time, searching for signs of why, but deep down I know it was me.

And then it happens again. I'm out running, crossing a road, convinced that I can get ahead of the car that's about to turn left across my path. I see it coming and suddenly decide to dodge it, but something is lost, some message between my brain and my legs fails to get through fast enough, and instead I stumble, falling flat on to the pavement again, this time thankfully bruising nothing more than my ego.

There are three of those falls in quick succession. The last time I land badly on my hand, and that afternoon, when I put my trainers away, something tells me it's for the last time. My brain and legs aren't talking to each other; the communication is lost. I go back to the doctor and there a nurse pulls blood from my veins into vials and sends them off.

'Everything is clear,' my GP tells me when I go back for the results, and again he mentions my age. I sit in front of him, unsure how to explain that everything is getting slower, that on bad days my mind can't instantly recall names and faces and places like it used to. Perhaps he is right and it is age, but I leave the surgery again with that impending sense of something I can't put my finger on, a sense that the doctor is missing something and yet I can't form enough thoughts to give him a clue as to what.

I remember the frantic pace, the speed with which you tackled things. I secretly admired that, even though I never would have said it. You drove everywhere, up and down the country all the time for work. On holidays you'd walk for miles across fells in the Lake District, right into the middle of nowhere, never minding if you got lost, because if you did, you had your wits about you – you would see distant landmarks, familiar sights and simply follow your nose. I couldn't do that. Not now.

We wouldn't get on now, you and I. Too much time has passed. We are friends who have lost touch, who now lead parallel lives. We like different things. You love the hustle and bustle of a busy city, whereas some days I lose hours just looking out of a window at the view. Just looking. Just still. And silent. But you always liked to be doing things, always wanted to be busy. You were never any good at just sitting. I have a lovely view where I live now. It's in a village not far from Beverley, East Yorkshire. Actually, you might remember — it's where Gemma lived. You fell in love with it too when we first came to visit, pointing out all the pretty red-brick cottages that line the street. You loved the friendly atmosphere, the fact everyone you met said hello whether they knew you or not. I do remember some things, like her showing you around the house, giving the guided tour, room to room, up and down stairs. You dutifully followed, excited too. Only she would have recognised that glint in your eye, that longing inside to roll your sleeves up and get stuck in, to open cans of paint and start decorating there and then. Nothing fazed you.

I am sitting in another hospital waiting room, with an overnight bag at my side purely as a precaution, or at least that's what I've told my eldest daughter Sarah, because I don't want her to worry. It had been the GP's idea to call one of my daughters when he handed me the referral letter, telling me to head straight to casualty. When I had phoned Sarah I'd promised there was nothing to panic about, that they would just need to check me over, that it would be nothing, although I'm not sure which one of us I was trying to convince. The sensation of a head half-filled with cotton wool has continued for months — since

9

the last fall – and this weekend it has been much, much worse. A fatigue that I couldn't fathom. My fork slipping from my hand, clattering on to my plate and into my dinner. When I got to work on Monday, my colleague noticed how my words slurred from my mouth, and she'd sent me home. It was clear that this was something much more serious than simply burning the candle at both ends. And now I'm here, sitting side by side with Sarah on the hard plastic hospital benches, looking out at the scene unfolding in front of us.

Sarah is still in the throes of her nursing training and her newly acquired medical eye roams over each patient as the pair of us observe other bodies in the room; the crude slings, the blood-soaked tea towels grabbed hurriedly, toddlers impatient to wait their turn, and the mothers trying hard to disguise their worry from them. The referral letter in my hand feels damp beneath my touch. When I'd shown it to the nurse who assessed me on arrival, I'd been surprised that she'd recognised my name as a patient, that the GP had already phoned ahead. Despite the fact that I knew the drill, that I work in hospitals, I didn't expect it to be happening to me.

They want to keep me in for monitoring. They're not sure what's to blame for the slurring, or at least even if they are, they haven't said. I'm sent back to the plastic chairs while I wait for a bed, and it's then that I convince Sarah not to wait with me.

'It could be hours yet,' I tell her. 'There's no point in us both sitting here.'

I see the doubt in her eyes, but she finally gathers up her coat and bag, and I promise to call her as soon as there is any news.

I was right to make her leave because it is hours later that they find me a bed. Darkness hangs outside at the windows as I'm led up to the ward. I lie on top of the sheets, still in the work clothes I'd dressed myself in that morning. All around me, nurses flit back and forth, never enough time between beds and patients, time flying on their shift, where for me it drags painfully. Ironically, I hate hospitals. I know I make a terrible patient. There's an electronic roster on the screen I can just make out from my bed and the nurses who buzz around have no idea that I can read from it just how understaffed they are, that I know whose feet are tired from the day shift, who's just arrived for the night. There's nothing to do but stare at the screen between checks until a nurse arrives to assess me more thoroughly.

'How long has your speech been affected?' she asks.

'I didn't know it was until this morning,' I tell her, as she takes a pen from her pocket.

'Can you pull me towards you?' she says, taking my weaker left arm in hers. I sense in her eyes that my arm is refusing to obey a simple test.

'OK, now push me away,' she says. The same again; she scribbles something on my notes, then leaves my bedside. I'm lucky tonight. They've put me into a side room, nothing to watch except different shades of blue as nurses hurry between beds outside. I slip into my pyjamas, but I don't sleep, the strange sounds from the machines I'm wired up to providing an unfamiliar soundtrack. Each time I feel my body relax, attempting to sink further into an unyielding mattress, an alarm goes off as my heart rate dips, a nurse rushes in and checks the screen, but I don't panic. I have a low resting heart rate; I'm fit and healthy. Aren't I?

You weren't the kind of person who forgot anything. Months or even years could go by and you would remember the name of someone you'd met just once. Your work colleagues were amazed by your recollection of anything: a case study, a file, a meeting. You always had an answer, despite the fact that technology was never your forte. You were good at your job — a non-clinical team leader in the NHS — that's why you threw everything into it, that's why you were such a workaholic. You managed rosters for hundreds of nurses, keeping all that information stored in your head. Everything was instantly available in your mind, and you never jumbled any of it up.

Which seems ironic now.

Your home life had been just as frantic as a busy single mum to two girls. Juggling all those balls in the air: a job, a house, two girls at school, no one to help. It seems a small wonder that none of those balls had dropped before. All the houses you bought needed doing up; you were always after another challenge. You never panicked. Within weeks, paper would be stripped, walls painted, and a brambly garden cut back to reveal a lawn long since hidden. Shrubs would be planted, seeds would be sown. Everywhere you moved you unintentionally left behind you a long list of henpecked husbands next door nagged by their wives for not sorting out their own DIY projects as quickly as you did yours. It was hard, but there was always a way; that was your motto. You liked a challenge, especially if it proved others wrong who thought you would never cope.

Maybe that's something we still have in common, and that gives me some comfort, that we still have some likenesses.

The next few days are taken up with tests and scans. I'm taken in a wheelchair through familiar corridors I once worked in, corridors I remember striding down confidently with colleagues, and I close my eyes and pray I won't be spotted by familiar faces. In different rooms, blood is pulled from my veins and arteries, and I watch doctors assess the results, wrinkling their noses and narrowing their eyes as if the little vial in front of them might give up the answer. The word 'stroke' is bandied between nurses and doctors, but nothing is confirmed and so I'm returned each time to a bed on the stroke ward beside patients who lie flat, unable to move or even speak, just a blank ceiling for company. I watch as the woman in the bed across from me attempts to use her stronger arm to reach out for her drink; her hand wobbles, overtaken by tremors in her attempt to get to the water. I look around, but all the nurses are busy with other patients, so I lift myself out of my bed and pass her the drink, feeling for a moment less helpless than I have for days, and at the same time an overwhelming feeling washes over me that I don't belong here, that I belong on the other side of the clipboard.

I want to leave now. I want to go home and put on my work clothes and return to my office, not be stuck here as a patient at the mercy of consultants too busy to give me more than five minutes of their time. Life as we know it has little bearing in here; what we thought of as a future has no certainty as we wait, for a nurse, a doctor, a scan, a test. There's a lot of time to think, to compare and contrast. At work you go about life looking forward to the weekend, wishing each Monday to Friday away; here there is nothing to do but watch and wait and think and worry, and wish back all those weeks that whizzed past, all those weeks of full fitness and a future stretched far ahead.

I watch the nurses turn the woman in the bed opposite me and wonder if she has accepted her lot as easily as it appears, or if she's just complying, waiting to be returned to the life she knows better but has unknowingly already kissed goodbye. I close my eyes and long for visiting time, when normal conversations can resume, when you can hear what's going on in the outside world, where routine means independence and a life fully lived, although those visiting us don't appreciate it, just like we forgot to. I see daughters stare at their mothers or fathers in beds before them, a shadow of the person who cradled them in their arms and wiped their tears when they cried, and I dread the day when my daughters might look at me like that. A student doctor arrives later that day and lingers longer over my notes; he looks down at me, asking how I'm feeling, not constrained by the strict regime enforced on his seniors. He has time to chat, to explain test results, to speculate over why no doctor has been able to confirm any diagnosis, and by the time he leaves my bed, I begin to feel more human again.

Today, as a last resort, I am being sent for a scan of my heart.

'Would you mind if a student carried out the procedure?' I'm asked. 'With the full supervision of a specialist, of course.'

I don't mind, and I'm pleased I agree, because as he moves the scanner up and down across my chest, he whispers his findings to his superior.

'Hole in the heart. It's quite common; it may have been the cause of the stroke,' the doctor says. And so with that, they seem happy to have some kind of explanation. Now thoughts turn to discharging me, and I'm returned to my bed on the ward with a hole in my heart but happy to be heading home.

Later that afternoon a physiotherapist appears at my bedside. They want to be sure that I will be able to manage at home with a left arm so slow and sluggish to receive signals from my brain. I'm taken to a mock-up kitchen off the ward, and it takes all my strength not to roll my eyes through the whole process of 'making' a cup of tea. Next the physio walks me up and down stairs while I cringe inside, and then I'm told that I'm ready to leave.

'I'm sorry we're still no clearer as to what caused the stroke,' the doctor who hands me my discharge papers says. 'But we've requested an outpatient's appointment with a neurologist, so that might get to the bottom of things.'

But it doesn't matter to me that things aren't adding up, and any problems I'd mentioned I'd been having with my memory seemed to have disappeared under a mound of other paperwork. I just want to leave, to return to my normal life, recover my certainty that everything is, in fact, OK.

I'm not used to being off work, so the only way I cope is by being creative with my recovery. The rain pouring down outside inspires me to devise my own exercises to strengthen my weak left arm, so I grab an umbrella and practise putting it up and down several times a day. At first the catch inches up the metal so slowly, my arm refusing to obey orders from my brain, but as the days go by it gets higher and higher until *click*, it slots into place and I stand there, alone in my living room, underneath a fully opened umbrella, wondering when I might be well enough to be back in the office.

The next two months at home drag. Each day I wonder how much more daytime television I can take before I risk exposing myself to another stroke. The Post-it note pad beside my bed sits unused, a reminder of my under-active brain. When I was in the office each day, I'd often wake up in the night, scrawl some reminder on a Post-it note and let it flutter down to the carpet as I went back to sleep, sure to feel it underfoot in the morning when I swung my legs over the side of the bed, unpeel it from the sole of my foot and instantly remember what I needed to do when I got to the office. But these days when I wake up and glance over the side of the bed, I'm met with nothing but the blankness of my pale green carpet. I used to curse the volume of Post-it notes scattered on the floor each morning, a symbol of the busy day ahead, and yet now how I long for just one single splash of pale yellow to tell me I still have a purpose.

I know busy life is continuing: I'm just not a part of it. I miss the team camaraderie that used to fill my day. I miss the buzz and working to deadlines. I used to wonder what it would be like to be retired, to do all those things I never had time for, and yet now I lack the energy or the inclination. But I've noticed something else too: as the date of returning to work comes closer, I start to doubt myself in a way I never have before. *What if I don't know what I'm doing any more?* The thought crosses my mind several times a day and I blink it away as if it never happened. Days pass and it's there again, and other doubts join it each morning, as if they breed overnight in my subconscious mind. *What if too much has changed? What if I can't remember the system? What if I become the one lagging behind, holding up everyone else?* I go back to my GP and tell him my fears, he reassures me that it's perfectly normal.

'Take another couple of weeks off to make sure you're really ready,' he says, and I'm surprised how willingly the sick certificate slots into my hand.

It is March 2013 — three months since the stroke — and I am back at work. Today is the first day, and as I re-familiarise myself with my desk, I look up and catch one of my colleagues watching me. He smiles but quickly looks away, and I turn back to my desk to start again, convinced he, too, is wondering if I can still do it. I turn on my computer, the screen blinks into life, and for a split second the desktop looks completely unfamiliar. I scan the various documents and files, looking for some point of reference and as the seconds tick by I feel my heart speed up in my chest. But there it is: the roster system. I double click, it opens up, and suddenly it all comes back to me. Of course I can do this.

The days go by as they always did, and even though maybe I creak rather than leap back into action, my confidence gathers as the weeks pass. The things I do forget — names or numbers, places, people — well, that's understandable. After all, I've been off for nearly three months, or at least that's what everyone around me says, and I start to believe it myself. Almost.

The neurology appointment comes through two months later, and I sit in front of the consultant trying to pinpoint the vagueness I've been feeling for months. What sense would it make to her if I explained that the pile of pale yellow Post-it notes scattered on the carpet had got thicker and thicker, as I woke numerous times in the night, desperate not to let a single thought slip through the net, remembering all I'd need to get through a day in the office.

'My mind just doesn't feel … sharp,' is all I could offer, and the consultant nods and writes down some notes in front of me. She prods and pokes around with more questions, but my answers come back woolly and vague.

'I'd like to refer you to a clinical psychologist,' she says. 'She'll be able to carry out more in-depth memory tests.'

I nod, a mixture of relief and concern that at last this is being given some attention. They run blood tests too, but as before, nothing shows up.

A month later, the clinical psychologist, Jo, introduces herself to me, and from the other side of the desk hands me three words that I'll need to remember during our session, and say to her once we've finished.

'OK,' I nod. It sounds simple enough.

Just like the neurologist, she asks me to describe the clouded thoughts I've been experiencing, trying her best to pinpoint when it started, how long it's been going on, whether it comes in waves or it's always there. I tell her about the ever-increasing pile of Post-it notes, in case it means anything to her; she nods as I say this and scribbles it down in her notes, and I feel it makes sense, as if it's relevant somehow. At the end of the session she closes her notebook and folds her arms across her chest.

'Now, can you tell me those three words I asked you to remember at the beginning of the session?' she says.

I stop, my eyes rolling up to the top of my head as if searching the archives above and yet failing to pull anything from them.

'I …' I shake my head. 'I'm sorry.'

She smiles. 'It's OK, don't worry, we've been talking about lots of different things.' She clears her throat. 'You're an intelligent, resourceful woman, Wendy, I can see that, and so I understand this confusion must be frustrating for you.'

'Is there anything I should do to help myself?' I say. 'In the times when my mind feels particularly … foggy.'

'Don't panic,' she says. 'There may come times when you become disorientated, the fog will descend and your surroundings will be unfamiliar, but the most important thing to remember is not to panic, give the fog time to pass, let the world become clear again. And it will.'

'OK,' I say. 'That makes sense.'

'What I recommend is we meet again in twelve months and see how things are for you then,' she says, her smile putting my mind at ease as she pulls a date from her diary. I get up to leave, still desperately trying to recall those three words as I cross her office, but as I go to close the door behind me, I notice that she's reopened my file and is writing something down inside.

As I make my way home, I go over the exercises I've just completed, like I've just left an exam and I'm trying to work out whether I've passed or not. Did I join up all the right dots, count the right shapes, draw the correct lines, and produce the right words? Did this brain I've known my whole life let me down?

I'm sitting opposite Sarah while she holds a letter in her hand, a letter from Jo after our last meeting. I scan her face as her eyes do the same to the page, taking it all in, not missing a single line, the clinical-speak making more sense now she's a few months further into her nursing training. I can tell just from watching her how far through the letter she is; she's currently reading the bit where Jo has detailed how independent I am, how well I manage at home, how organised I am. But then she turns the page and I see her brow furrow and I remember the moment when my own did the same. It's one line below a heading that says 'Opinion' in thick, bold type. She looks up and I catch her eye.

'Dementia?' she says.

But that isn't what it says. I know exactly what it says. I've burned it into my memory. *It is possible that this is a profile of the early stages of a dementing process.*

Sarah puts the letter down. 'But it can't be that,' she says. 'You're so fit and healthy. It doesn't seem fair.'

I know, I've been thinking the same thing since I tore open the envelope myself.

I take a breath. 'Exactly,' I say. 'I'm sure it's nothing like that, but I suppose they have to cover every eventuality.' But I can already see the worry that's cast a spell over Sarah's face, as if her eyes are windows to the exact same images that are swimming around in my own head when it comes to dementia patients: white-haired, old people in beds, unable to recognise their own children, or to remember their own names.

'It could be a million other things,' I say, putting the letter back in the envelope. Because that's what I've told myself: the word was 'possible' and within it is so much room for doubt.

A few weeks later, there's another letter, this time from the neurologist. Both of my girls are here to read it: *To be certain* [of this representing an early dementia] *we would need to demonstrate deteriorating cognition in six to twelve months' time. If no change I would diagnose mild cognitive impairment,* writes the neurologist. *However, if there is a definite deterioration then the diagnosis would be dementia.*

The three of us sit quietly, and I look across the living room at my two girls, now grown women, though often still little girls in my eyes. That's nothing to do with my memory or whatever it is that's afflicting my brain, that's the lens a mother always views her children through; no matter how old they get, or how tall they grow over us, the urge to protect them never dims. But I know these two faces as well as my own, and the telltale signs of worry that flash across them, the secret giveaways: the fleeting stare from the youngest that has always meant she's frightened inside, but she'd never say, not even as a child. The hint of a frown and quiver in the voice of the eldest, who's always been less able to hide her fears. So I don't even blink for fear of missing a reaction, and there it is on both of them. I push down the guilt that reaches up from my gut.

'There's no point in worrying,' I say breezily, standing up to make a cup of tea. 'There's nothing we can do but wait for the summer when they do more tests. What's the point in worrying until we have something to worry about?'

It feels as if my words are avoiding something, and as I leave the room it comes to me: fear.

You never liked your girls to worry. Did it make you feel more vulnerable that there was only you to worry for them? You would never have said so; you kept your fears to yourself. I can still see

24

you now in the ward, sitting up in the hospital gown that had been hastily slipped around your shoulders two hours previously, the lick of brown iodine still dyeing your flesh beneath it, and yet you told yourself you were well enough to make a phone call. You put on your best and bounciest voice; you dialled home to check everything was OK. That instinct to be Mum overpowering the last of the general anaesthetic still running through your veins.

You hadn't felt well that morning, but you'd gone to work anyway; you hated letting anyone down. The girls were at secondary school then, and you'd only allowed the stomach pain inside to bite once you'd seen them off in their freshly pressed navy uniforms. It was harder to hide it at work though, that tiny film of sweat settling on your brow. You sat behind the desk where you worked as a hospital receptionist, putting patients' health before your own, telling yourself and anyone else who asked that you were fine. But as the day went by, the pain crept from your left-hand side to your face for all to see. It was almost 3 p.m., the end of the school day, by the time the registrar in casualty came to take a look at you. He quickly started talking about emergencies and operating theatres; he wouldn't listen when you said you were fine, you just needed to be home by the time the girls left school. Your appendix wouldn't wait that long. Even as the anaesthetist asked you to count backwards you were telling yourself that your friend lived nearby if there was an emergency. Missing the fact that you were the one in danger.

You awoke, minus the inflamed appendix, and tried to move, wincing in pain. But then you thought of the girls and the guilt that they had no one but you made your heart ache in a way that overwhelmed the raw wound in your side. It took all your strength to roll out of bed, to shuffle down the corridor to the ward phone clutching the 10p pieces you'd been lucky enough to have in your purse. The relief when you heard their voices was matched only by the throbbing underneath your National Health gown, which hastened you back to bed. You lay there smiling. It was excitement, not fear, you heard in their voices, a sense of adventure and responsibility, of fending for themselves. But wasn't that how you'd always brought them up? To manage alone, as you had to.

All pain was removed from your face in preparation for their visit the following day. They chattered excitedly about how they'd managed without you and you nodded and smiled, grateful for friends who'd helped out. They were only eleven and fourteen, yet they wouldn't leave your side before hearing for themselves from the consultant that you were getting better, that you'd soon be home, that when you told them you were OK you meant it. Perhaps there have always been giveaway clues of fear in your face too. Perhaps that's why you understand their need to know everything now.

I've been staring at the same computer screen for the last twenty minutes and it still makes little sense. I have tentatively tried tapping various keys and yet nothing's happened, or at least not what I wanted to. I have two screens open, one with the old system that I know so well, the other the new system that we need to get to grips with. But something isn't clicking. I might as well be staring at a foreign language. I close the screen, frustrated, tell myself I'll tackle it again tomorrow, but I said the same yesterday. Instead I'll do what I did last night, try again with the remote access I have at home, so no one sees the extra hours I'm putting in just to keep up. It has been six months since my appointment with Jo and the world is no clearer than it was then. Today we have a meeting about the new computer system for the rosters. It is my job to tell the managers and matrons how the plans are going for the rollout, and yet it remains a mystery to me. It's something that at one time I would have got in an instant, but now I'm the one creating delays that shouldn't exist.

A few hours later I'm in the meeting room, sitting at a conference table, faces looking at me expectantly while I explain the new system and its benefits, despite the fact I'm still to fully comprehend them myself. I glance around the table at faces I know are familiar, and yet I can't recall their names, and this little internal fear, this tiny seed of worries whittles away inside until I'm shuffling my paperwork, confused about where to start. It's my turn to speak. I look up.

'We expect to start rolling out the system in two months' time …' I pause, every eye upon me, but the word I need next is lost, and instead there is a blank in my mind where it should be. The silence hangs in the room and for a fraction of a second I'm sure I see the questions behind their eyes, wondering if I am fit for this job, why I can't complete a simple sentence. I feel stupid then. Stupid, frustrated, confused, humiliated. It's a moment that seems to last for ever. Perhaps it was only a second, but the word I need eludes me and so I look down at the paperwork for inspiration, starting somewhere else, hoping I've glanced over the heavy pause.

'W—we've had a few glitches, but most of the data has been easy to transfer.'

An hour later, the meeting finishes and people file from the room. I linger, picking up my paperwork from the desk, and then it comes to me, the word I'd been so desperately searching for. I look up quickly, as if other people might have spotted the moment of recognition on my face, at the same time as I swallow down the shame, because the word I had been so desperately racking my brain for was something tiny, something simple. It was 'and'.

An appointment for a SPECT scan arrives in April 2014. It's a 3D scan of my brain, which the neurologist says may prove more helpful than the MRI.

'We're going to inject this dye into your vein and that way we can monitor how it travels through your brain,' the radiologist says.

I lie back in a dimly lit room, alone in my thoughts as the dye makes its way around my brain, although I don't feel a thing. The nurse tells me that I can sleep as I lie here, but I am determined to stay awake and alert, as if somehow my brain and I can trick the system into finding it anything but sluggish. Deep inside I know, though, this type of camera never lies; the dye will seep through, finding the roadblock in my brain that is causing all this destruction. I feel again that helplessness I'm trying to get accustomed to, allowing the scans and tests to reveal more about my body than I'm able to articulate, but there's an image that keeps coming back to me of driving on a motorway at speed, the warning lights above the carriageway lighting up to warn of worsening conditions up ahead, going down through the gears, 60, 40, 20 mph, until the brake lights in front bring you to a halt altogether. Is that what it's like in my brain at the moment?

A few days later I'm driving in my car, and suddenly I'm aware of the car behind me. It feels close, imposing. I've always despised tailgaters, considered them incompetent and bad drivers. My hands grip the steering wheel. *Why is he making me feel so nervous when he is the problem?* I blink, narrow my eyes as I feel the need to concentrate, hunch forward in my seat. I look up at the road, but that's all I can do, simply look. *What do I do next?* Why won't the next process come into my head? A horn blares angrily behind me. I glance into my rearview mirror and see headlights flashing, an exasperated face behind the wheel. I wince, though I'm not sure why. I know this road, I've been down this residential street countless times before, so why is something missing? I just need a moment to work out what to do. I need to turn right at the end of the road, but how? How do I turn right? My brain will only process one action at a time, yet I see signs, markings on the road. I know I need to move, but it's all merging together, becoming a tangled mess in my mind. Another blast of the horn behind me. My hands grip the wheel tighter. I glance down at the dashboard and I understand why the car behind is flashing: the speedometer is wavering somewhere around 10 mph. How did that happen? Still the junction is approaching too quickly. I can't think in time. Another beep. Flashing lights. I cringe. I turn left instead of right, away from my destination. The car behind me has gone, but my skin is tingling, panicked. My breath is short. I'm lost inside. *I couldn't process it quick enough. My brain and my body weren't talking*, I think.

I pull over and lean over the steering wheel. I close my eyes, take deep breaths, but I don't feel safe. *Why couldn't I turn right?*

I wait and wait at the side of the road. 'You can do this,' I say to myself inside my silver Suzuki Swift.

The traffic zooms by, everyone else going about the everyday, rushing here and there on automatic; nothing has changed for them. But the metaphorical roadblock I'd been imagining days before is real now.

Finally, I take a deep breath and turn the key in the ignition. 'You've been driving all your life, Wendy,' I tell myself.

I flick the indicator right, check the dashboard to make sure it's on, listen for the comforting *click-click*. I check my mirror, over my shoulder, everything exaggerated. Check once, check again, more like a learner than someone who has been driving for thirty-three years. *I just want to be home.* Slowly, I pull out on to the road, holding tight on to every nerve until I see my street approaching. I let out a sigh of relief as I pull the handbrake up to stop.

A few days later I get into the car again. I manage to calm the heart beating wildly beneath my seat belt, taking a moment to familiarise myself with my surroundings; indicators, gears, handbrake, as if I'd never done this before. I'd always just jumped into my car without much thought. Hadn't I been the woman who had driven all over the country, who found her way anywhere long before satnavs? The other day had been a blip. I set off along straight roads and feel my confidence return as the speedometer rises higher: 20, 30, 40. I turn left, straighten up, another left turn. No problem. I begin to relax and then there's a right turn ahead; the speedometer dips, taking my confidence with it. I glance in the rearview mirror, look back at the road ahead, my feet not talking to my brain, the car over-revving, my hand fumbling with the gears. It's happening again. Only one process can filter through at a time. *There's not enough time to think how to turn right.* A different me clutches the wheel, hands clammy; it slips beneath my grasp.

I made it home that day, and put my keys down in their usual place, in a red dish on the hall table by the stairs. They sat there, looking back at me whenever I passed.

Useless, nonfunctional, incompetent, idle.

The piece of paper Sarah has put on the table in front of us looks like it has a giant spider drawn on it in black biro. A giant spider with 'Mum' written on its belly, shaded lightly with yellow as if, perhaps, to lighten the subject. I stare at it for a moment, at the spindly legs and all the words in fat bubbles on the end of each one: living/housing, anxiety, interests, and finally, Sarah. I can see how much effort she's put into this brainstorming diagram, an outline of all the thoughts she's about to explain to me. But what I really want to do is to close my eyes, to turn the piece of paper over, to stay in the life I know rather than the new one sketched out on the table in front of us.

'I've tried to put on to paper how I'm feeling ...' she starts. 'I want you to know you can rely on me.'

I don't have to look up to know her face will be turned slightly away from mine until she is sure she's on safe ground, and it's in that moment that I switch from patient to mother. I paste a smile on to my face for her to see, suffuse my voice with that subtle encouraging inflection, the same one that, decades before, had urged each of my girls to try a new word out loud to me from a book at bedtime or spill secrets that were troubling them. And I listen, even though I don't want to. I do it for her.

'I think these are some of the things that we may need to think about if the diagnosis does turn out to be dementia ...' I hear the hesitation in her voice, and in turn try to disguise the fear in mine and listen as she talks me through the diagram, growing more confident as she does. She hovers over each of the little bubbles. I see she's written *stairs?* and then crossed it out, and I think of my running shoes in the back of the wardrobe, the same ones I haven't slipped my feet into for months.

Her finger darts across the diagram. As it does, my gaze lingers on the word *care*, and something tightens deep inside. I'm not ready for this, and yet she needs to talk, she needs to explore all those what-ifs, and I need to listen. It's what mums do. It's a strange conversation, the past, present and future versions of ourselves colliding. Sarah shows me around her diagram proudly; she wants me to know she's capable, that she can manage, that I – in turn – will be able to manage. The writing is neat, the diagram well drawn, and I think back for a second to other drawings she'd run out of school clutching, eager to show me, and I feel that same sense of pride at my daughter's practical brain despite the subject matter.

'OK,' I say when she's finished. 'I'll have a think about this and get back to you.'

A flicker of hurt crosses her face, momentary, something only I would notice. She wants decisions, conclusions, worst-case scenarios addressed; it'll make her feel better, more in control of what's going on inside my head or what the doctors might find. But I can't do it for her, I'm just not ready.

'We don't even know if there will be a dementia diagnosis,' I say. 'Some of the things you've written down are way in the future—'

'But—'

'It's too soon to think about them now.'

I don't mean it to come out so abrupt. I try a different voice. 'I just don't want to talk about dementia any more until we have a diagnosis.'

'OK, Mum,' she soothes.

The roles reversed again. We change the subject. She stops sending me links to dementia articles.

A few days later another email lands in my inbox. My finger hovers over the mouse before I click 'open'. If I do, am I colluding with this disease? Am I inviting it into my inbox, my home, my head? I'd wondered the same when I'd typed out my initial enquiry.

'*Thank you for contacting the Alzheimer's Society ...*' it starts. My heart is racing at the secret I've kept from the girls. I read the email quickly, as if it's sent from an illicit lover, my eyes scanning for sweet nothings, my finger ready to click it closed if anyone appears by my side. And then I find it, an answer to my question: a dementia diagnosis would entitle me to a free bus pass. I lean in closer, read again.

Footsteps in the hall make me snap the screen shut, Sarah waking up and walking in.

The morning goes by and I'm still thinking of that bus pass. The first positive thing I've read. My brain in exchange for a bus pass. A ludicrous swap.

If I close my eyes I can still see you, always with a paint roller in your hands, sleeves rolled up, the same white shirt splattered with years of paint, black jogging bottoms speckled with colours of rooms over the years; the sky-blue bathroom in Annesley Road, the deep-red feature wall at Dolben Court, every single sunshine-yellow kitchen. The Beatles' White Album *spinning on the record player, having to put down your brush and dry your hands on a rag to turn it over. The scissors always glided through the paper perfectly, quickly, effortlessly, every pattern matched, never too much wasted, each bubble smoothed out from the wall before the glue had time to set. You worked fast, singing while you hung wallpaper or painted walls; footsteps on the stairs, the girls running in and out to ask what time tea was ready, where a certain book or toy might be.*

I took your independence for granted then. I envy it now.

First I switch the Beatles off, hearing the gentle whirring sound inside the hi-fi as the CD comes to a halt. It's annoying having to keep stopping and starting to press play again anyway, I reason. I go back to the pasting table and take a deep breath: where was I? I'm decorating my home office, a busy pattern of tiny red roses running down ivy – it had reminded me of a bouquet of barbed wire in the shop. I try again, look from the roll of paper to the wall, but the pattern swims in front of my eyes, I can't see the obvious place to cut and when I do, the scissors inch through, tearing jagged lines into the paper. I roll my eyes, start again, and again, and soon I've wasted half a roll of paper. Finally I get it on to the pasting table, trying to ignore the creases I've made in the paper. The paste splatters on the floor, and I trip as I carry it to the wall. But I've forgotten where the pattern matches, and the seam isn't pushed up to the paper hung before it, so a thin line of magnolia goads me the whole way down the wall, huge bubbles caught underneath. I drop the brush on the floor at my feet in frustration, and tear the slimy paper from the wall. I go back to the pasting table and start again.

I can do this. I've done it dozens of times before.

But the hours have passed and outside the night is black, the clock creeping towards twelve. I'll try again tomorrow.

I hesitantly peer round the corner of the door into the home office the following morning, mug in hand; I swallow down the shame of the mess on the walls along with my Yorkshire tea. The wallpaper isn't even straight: the bubbles of air trapped underneath distort the pattern. If I didn't need to be at work, I'd scrape it all down now.

I try again that night, and the next. Every piece that should sit snug and seamless is now accompanied by a streak of magnolia beneath. I know I used to look forward to papering around sockets, getting the paper to fit seamlessly. Now too much paper is snipped away, wildly overestimated, a mess.

It's nothing more than my ego that keeps me in that tiny room for three evenings, wasting more paper and paste, unable to understand the following morning why the pattern hangs skew-whiff. I'd done it to prove the doctors wrong, to rubbish what was in those letters, to prove to Sarah I didn't need brainstorming diagrams, to show the neurologist that we weren't looking at a decline. I was going to outwit any impending diagnosis; I *was* still capable. But in the end I was left with nothing but three evenings of continued failure. Proving nothing more to myself than my new inability. I switch off the light and close the door. I know I won't try again.

A few weeks later, I wake and sit on the edge of my bed, looking down at my feet. Where once there was pale green carpet, there is a crunch of yellow Post-it notes between my toes. The pile has grown thicker after another restless night of waking, turning, remembering something else I'll need for the next day, my confidence at each thought surviving sleep fading with each dark hour that went by. I glance at my alarm clock: 4.50 a.m., the same time I've been waking for work for years, ready and out the door for the first bus at 5.35 a.m. I bend over and unpeel a few Post-its from under my heels; by the time I look up again, it is 5 a.m.; ten minutes lost, how did that happen? I need to move, but I can't think what I do first. Dress? Eat? Shower? No, that doesn't feel right. I look beyond the curtains, momentarily confused by the sleep still soft between my ears and the dark clouds outside. I glance at the clock again to check it's definitely morning.

After a while, I head to the bathroom, and it's thirty minutes later by the time I'm dressed and downstairs. I switch breakfast TV on, a routine I know so well, but I stare at the clock on the screen, confused. It's 5.30 a.m. – I should be at the bus stop by now, but I've only just poured a cup of tea. Time running through my fingers like sand, I grab my coat and bag and hurry from the house.

I make the bus, but I'm hot and flustered. I sit in my usual seat on the top deck for the best view; at this time in the morning the bus is empty, so it's all mine. There's a still sky at the windows, the rest of the world is yet to wake; even the birds still sleep in the trees, and I'm retracing my steps, wondering where I lost time again today.

At work I turn on my computer and the log-in screen flashes up. I stare at it for a second longer than I know I should, wondering what it's asking from me. When I type in my details, the screen opens up and it takes me a few moments to make sense of it, the same desktop I've been greeted by for years feeling more like I'm seeing it for the first time.

I've still managed to arrive at my desk an hour earlier than everyone else. I used to use the time in a deserted office to get ahead for the day, but now I pull the pile of sticky notes from my handbag and work through them one by one, screwing each one into a tiny ball when I'm done and burying it in the bottom of the waste-paper bin. There are days when the fog feels heavier than others. On those days when I open the roster system, the coloured squares that make perfect sense on any other day swim in front of my eyes, meaningless. On those days, I dread the knock on my office door, a head peering round the corner, or a body appearing beside my desk with a question. I know that there will be a blank written large across my face. I know that I'll try to distract them from it, shuffling papers on my desk, making an excuse that I need to be somewhere else.

Answering the phone on days like that has become more and more difficult. It had always been such a natural part of my job, my number almost a helpline to worried ward sisters, yet now I know instinctively that their fears are not assuaged by the hesitancy in my voice when I pick up their call. Instead of their concerns, other more distracting thoughts are whirring round my brain: *Why are they talking so fast? Can't they speak more slowly to give me time to think?* I ask again what the problem is, cringing inwardly at the slight sigh they let fall down the receiver, knowing it must appear to them that it's someone else on the end of the line, not the person they've come to rely on. I have become a master of disguise, of buying time, and so I suggest they come into the office to discuss the problem, I tell them that it would be nice to see them, that it will be easier to show them in person, or I'll visit them on the ward. A delaying tactic. Not a lie but a more convenient truth, because the phone, with its faceless voices, has become an enemy. Faceless voices don't see the concentration on your face, they don't know you're searching the Rolodex in your mind for answers. Faceless voices get impatient, they bombard you with more questions, they are demanding, they unwittingly add to the confusion that reigns.

Those days are becoming more and more frequent, the focus fading as the months pass, the lens softening from crystal clear to something just a little more blurred, which has become my new normal. Not that I've told anyone – not at work, anyway; instead I find more ways to cover up the problems, but there are times when I simply can't camouflage the confusion. The meetings when I struggle to put a name to the person who is smiling at me across the table, a colleague I know I've met before, missing the conversation because I'm sifting through it for the mention of a name, or reading the notes she has in front of her for a clue. There's the panic when people I've worked with for years walk into the room and a blank meets my mind, a space inside where their name usually fitted neatly and I see that flicker of doubt reflected in their own faces, which makes my heart race under my shirt. There was the sister I know so well who called me to visit her on the ward; her name and voice had meant nothing to me on the phone, and it was only when I arrived there that I realised we were friends.

'I thought I'd done something to offend you!' she'd said.
And I laughed it off, blaming a busy day.
But I'm running out of excuses.

As another day draws to a close, I switch off my computer and gather up my things. I walk the two miles from the hospital to the bus station, and find my regular seat upstairs, the same one from which I watched the world wake this morning. Only on this journey home, I am exhausted. The bus ride takes just over an hour, as the landscape changes from city to countryside, the walls that hug York itself turning into hedges that wrap around fields. My heavy eyelids close, enjoying the nothingness that sleep brings. But I wake with a start, sitting up and looking around to get my bearings, terrified I might have missed my stop. Am I heading to the Scarborough coast? By the time I see my stop just in sight, making my wobbling descent down the stairs, I'm longing for the safety of home, the solitude, the peace, the non-taxing television and its mindless programmes. I've survived another day. And yet tomorrow the challenges I faced today might be even harder.

Six months later I'm sitting in front of Jo again as she tells me the three words she wants me to remember by the end of the session. She starts going through the same memory tests as she did six months ago. When she asks me to name objects beginning with a certain letter, nothing comes. I glance around the room for inspiration, my eyes flicking back to hers, noticing how she watches me, how she knows I'm cheating.

'Take your time,' she says gently.

Eventually I find a pen, a pad, a pencil.

'OK,' she says, writing them down.

It's obvious to both of us that there has been a decline, and yet Jo's gentle, confident manner distracts from the fear that's gathering in the pit of my stomach. She leans across the desk and hands me a piece of paper and a pen.

'Can you draw a clock for me?' she says.

Easy, I think, and yet when I lean forward, the pen hovers above the paper; the circle isn't quite what I remember a circle looking like. I start filling in the numbers, my brow furrowed in concentration, but it doesn't look right – the twelve is in the wrong place. I sit back and stare at the page. Why is there no room for the twelve?

'I'm sorry,' I say. 'It's so strange. It's just a clock.'

'It's OK,' she says, making another scribble inside her notes. And then she asks for those three words she'd told me at the beginning of the session, and again, they've slipped away without me noticing.

'We've got two more weeks to go, Wendy,' she smiles, closing my file. 'Plenty of time to try again.'

The third and final set of test days dawns and I'm back in front of Jo as we go through similar tests and this time, it's just the same. At the end of our session, she sits back in her chair.

'How do you think that went?' she says.

'I know it didn't go well,' I venture. I pause for a second, enough time to muster up the question I've wanted to ask for so many months. 'What do you think it could be?' I say finally.

She looks into my eyes, and her voice is calm and steady. 'Possibly dementia, but I can't be completely sure, not until we get the results of all the tests.'

'Of course,' I reply. But I'm not sure how the words reach my mouth because a numbness embraces me, and a sadness too, a feeling that this is the end because that's

all I know about dementia; the blank stares, the helplessness, the confusion. And everything I'd been determined
to avoid since I first saw whispers of the word in the
letters that went between Jo and my neurologist.

Back at home, I sit down in front of my computer,
open YouTube, and slowly type in the letters, my
finger hovering over the return key before I search for
'dementia', daring myself perhaps, unsure if I'm ready
to see the results. The videos that appear on screen are
exactly the images that my mind has been conjuring
up since Jo uttered the words; men and women at the
ends of their lives, old and white-haired, blankness
written large across every face, confined to hospital
beds. Surely she must have got it wrong? None of
these people are like me. My eyes skip through those
videos, searching for something else, something more
relatable and at the same time hoping that anything
like me doesn't appear, and that's when I find Keith
Oliver.

When the video starts, I'm relieved to see an intelligent man similar in age to me, sitting in a chair at home,
his backdrop a beautiful green garden, speaking lucidly
and eloquently into camera. As he starts to tell his story
– how he was the headteacher of a busy Canterbury
school, how two years before the recording he started
to have unexpected falls, a feeling of fatigue, of just feeling 'unwell' – I am transfixed. I watch more in utter

silence, mesmerised how, like me, he'd started to struggle at work with simple tasks like meeting deadlines, retrieving and recalling information, using the phone, multitasking. The more I watch, the more it makes sense, and yet the recognition is no longer frightening. Instead, a feeling of relief is creeping over me. He likens having dementia to the weather; some days are sunny, but on others the clouds gather. 'When it's a sunny day, I can hold a conversation with very little difficulty,' he explains. 'On a foggy day, finding those words is a real challenge.'

I think back to all the days at work when I've felt isolated in conversations, finding it impossible to retrieve the right words to join in or keep up. Keith has experienced exactly the same thing. His story was so positive: he talked about how he felt that his health had maintained a good level since his diagnosis thanks to his determination to live life to the full and focus on the things he enjoyed. By the time the eight-minute clip has come to an end, life really doesn't seem as bleak. The ideas I had about what a person with dementia looks and sounds like have been challenged. Keith looks so normal, and I must look no different; he still does the things he enjoys, and so I could, too. It's not so much mortality that hits me full on, but that sense of time – or, rather, lack of it. That's what dementia steals, the future you imagined all laid out in front of you, with no idea when something more final might come.

I go to sleep that night determined not to let the worry whittle away at me as I sleep, and yet I lie awake, blinking in the blackness, unable to push the dark thoughts that accompany that time of night from my mind. I'm fifty-eight years old and I face a diagnosis of dementia. Is it really that? Might the doctors be wrong? What are the chances? Over and over it goes until my brain wears itself out and sleep creeps up on me.

If I could ask you anything now, it would be: When did you decide to leave me? When did you decide that I was to live a different life without all the bits that made me me? It's hard to remember those final experiences of things I so enjoyed, like desperately trying to catch a drifting dream the next morning. I wish I had known then that they were the last times I would do those things I loved and I would have enjoyed them all the more for knowing: the last run along deserted streets, the last batch of cakes, the last drive behind the steering wheel. Instead you sneaked out on me, you didn't tell me you were going, and so I never knew you'd taken bits of me with you. You didn't give me a chance or warning, so I couldn't try and rescue those days. I simply discovered one day that they were gone, gone forever.

But if I had to pinpoint the moment you left, I know which day I would choose, the day I think you left me properly for the first time. Before that it had been a long goodbye; this was more like ripping a plaster off – it was fast, whipped away in a second. I looked up from my desk and you were gone, although I didn't know that then, because in that second, I had no memory of you. I had no memory of anything. It was like I had just arrived, had looked up and found myself in a place I'd never been to before, surrounded by strangers.

This day was different from any that had come before it. It wasn't just confusion. It was a complete blank. A black hole. It wasn't so much, What did I get up for? What was I about to do? *It was,* Where am I? *My mind was blank, my intention as confused as the speckles on the green linoleum beneath my feet. Where was I? What was this place? I felt my heart thumping with questions, pounding for answers from my brain. But nothing came. I stood and froze for a second. I tried again, my eyes flickering round this room; a desk, noticeboards pinned to the walls, box files scribbled with handwriting I didn't recognise. My heart rapped harder against my ribs and I replied with a long, deep breath, which quietened it for a brief moment. Another breath. It shushed inside. Something was cutting through the fog that had descended on my brain. One memory. Jo told me this would happen and she told me it would pass. And so I started walking, out of the office door and the desk I left behind. The room with the grey metal filing cabinet, and strange trinkets on a desk that I'd never seen before in my life. Past the name on* the door that I didn't recognise, the letters that formed them as alien as their meaning.

W-E-N-D-Y M-I-T-C-H-E-L-L.

I walked out into the hallway, looking straight ahead, resisting any urge to search the walls for clues, ignoring the paperwork that clung to them, knowing instinctively it would only add to the confusion. I avoided the glare of the wall lights, tried to block out the hum of voices I'd never heard before. I walked slowly, trying to concentrate on keeping my breath steady, on blocking out the laughter, resisting the urge to ask if they're laughing at me.

Don't panic, I told myself. Office doors were open either side of the corridor, inside the rooms, heads I didn't recognise looked down at paperwork. I dreaded them – whoever they were – looking up and being greeted by the blankness on my face, calling out to say hello and spotting the mystery I just knew would be there, etched across it. I didn't want anyone to speak to me, to pull me into their world, because I didn't know that world, I didn't know the people in it. A blank existed between me and them. And it could have terrified me if I let it. Instead I carried on walking, letting each foot take one step in front of the other, to where I didn't know. The tap of the floor underfoot breaking the silence around me, a slight antiseptic smell permeating my nose. There were double doors at the end of the corridor. I headed through them into a stairwell. Somewhere quieter, no people. There was another door with a faded, patterned-glass panel, and something told me it would offer sanctuary. The pale pink walls that greeted me were instantly calming. The emptiness of it, the isolation, the silence. I went into a cubicle, sat down on the closed toilet seat. And waited.

It felt like I was in there for hours, but there is no concept of time in moments like that. My brain was cloudy, a fog had descended, like the peak of Scafell Pike on a clear day where one minute I could see for miles, and then suddenly a chill in the air indicated the clouds were forming. Yet for me, there was no warning, no change in the temperature to show that change was coming. I'd got up from my desk just like any other day, and suddenly I was at the top of that mountain, alone, the clouds obscuring my view to such an extent that I couldn't see any landmarks I recognised, not my desk, nor my phone, my stapler, my name on the door, or even my colleagues. Not on that day in particular. And so I waited, because Jo's words were the only clarity in my mind. Just sit and hold on for the mist to clear. And so I did. In my tiny cubicle, my eyes flickering between the floor and the speckled pattern of the wall tiles, the toilet-roll holder and the sheet of two-ply that hung limply from it.

And then there it was. The cloud was lifting. I looked up as if I'd been dreaming. I was in the toilets at work. Of course I was.

Today's date is 31 July 2014. It has been embedded in my mind for weeks now for two reasons; firstly, it is the day that Sarah has planned to move out of my home and into the new home she will share with her boyfriend.

Secondly, it is the date I'm due to receive my diagnosis from the neurologist.

Sarah, Gemma and I haven't discussed the impending news in the last few days; it is an unspoken thing, a diagnosis we are all sure of, the deterioration predicted in earlier letters now clear for us all to see without the need for a medical eye. What is there left to discuss?

And so I am here at the hospital alone, sitting in the cramped office of the neurologist as she shuffles through the paperwork between us. As she starts to speak, I know that it isn't so much what she's saying that will stick firm in my mind, but the way she is looking at me, the pity so apparent in her eyes. She doesn't actually say much at all, and from the moment I was called into her tiny office she hasn't needed to, because I'd seen it for myself when I'd glanced down at the paperwork in front of her, before she picked it up: Alzheimer's. She's pointing at it now, along with another word – dementia – her pen is flipping between the two, she is telling me that this is the letter she will be sending to my GP. All I can wonder in this moment is why she's pointing out these two words to me. Is it to make it that bit clearer, to make sure I believe her? Is it because there's nothing on my face to signal that I'm taking it in? Only my eyes move as I stare at the paper in front of me. I am calm. There's nothing left to question; the answer is in front of me in black and white. Despite the video of Keith Oliver and all the positive things he said about dementia, nothing prepares you for a diagnosis of your own, for that feeling of emptiness, because I know these words, this letter, will change everything, they'll change the life I know. They'll *steal* the life I know. I'm fifty-eight years old, and I've just been diagnosed with young-onset Alzheimer's.

Or perhaps she is showing me those two words because she can see the blank gaze, because as she talks I'm picturing another letter in my mind. One I held in my hand a few weeks ago from the pension company, stating that I was due to retire at sixty-six. That leaves an eight-year deficit. How will I fill it? That's what's going through my mind: what will happen to me in the next eight years? How will life look? I see today's date at the top of her paperwork, and I think of Sarah about to embark on a new beginning, when this letter for me represents an ending. There is some relief there, an end to one type of uncertainty, a beginning of another.

'Good luck,' she says as I leave her office. I won't see her again, because there is no follow-up after diagnosis. There's nothing they can do.

I start the short walk home, watching others going about their daily routines, noting how life goes on around me, and yet at this moment, mine has come to a standstill. I know Sarah will be back at the house, packing the last of her boxes, pulling the last few clothes from hangers in her wardrobe. She will offer to stay with me, of course she will, but that's not what I want or need. She'd stayed with me during her nursing training – it had made better financial sense while she was a student – but it's not necessary now, she must become independent again, and today's diagnosis changes nothing. I close my eyes briefly and an image flashes into my head, as if the future has been fast-forwarded in my mind; I am in a bed, my hair grey, my daughter caring for me. I shake it away, along with a dozen other questions and images. I don't want my girls to become my carers. Why would I rid them of the title 'child' and label them with something else they don't want and didn't ask for? How could I allow their dreams to be put on hold to care for me?

I fish a pen from my bag and write on the back of the letter that the neurologist handed me: *From where I am now, what's the average time to deteriorate – what are the stages and things to look out for?*

I walk on automatically, questions coming too quickly to catch. Instead I quickly shut each one away in my mind behind a door and turn the key, afraid to let them run wild and out of control. I arrive home and let myself in, the neurologist's words still settling in my brain, not separated by enough space or time to cushion the blow to my girls, my breezy mum voice lost under the weight of worry. Sarah greets me in the hall, we exchange a glance before I say anything, and I see that instant where her shoulders drop just a millimetre.

'It was what we expected,' I say, my voice sounding detached and unfamiliar. The silence settles for a moment between us, and then I call Gemma and tell her the same.

We're here again at the hospital four weeks later. The girls had arrived at my place early to give us plenty of time to walk to the hospital, alleviating the stress of having to find a parking space. We'd walked together in silence, Sarah and Gemma holding tight on to their thoughts, most of them captured in notes written between them that I'd spotted sticking out of their handbags. I lead the way into the hospital, finding my way to the same row of hard green plastic seats I'd sat in myself a few weeks before. We sit in the waiting area together, one of the girls on each side of me, and I'm not sure who is protecting whom. Each time I hear footsteps, I glance up, until at last I see the familiar face of the neurologist.

I guide the girls into the room and make the introductions; there's the same desk where I sat just weeks before, the same bundle of paperwork, the same pitiful smile stuck fast to the consultant's face – all she can offer me. We'd agreed that I would leave them in the room alone as this meeting is to help them understand. I wanted them to be able to ask whatever questions they needed to without worrying how I might react, and so I leave and head back to the waiting area. As I sit there, I remind myself that they have each other in that room, and I know that if one of them stumbles on a question, the other will finish the sentence. I even picture the glances that will pass between them, lost on the neurologist perhaps, but they would have been so visible to me.

Outside there is a box of toys that seem long since abandoned. An abacus sits on top, painted in primary colours that have faded and dulled as the life has worn out of it. I picture Gemma and Sarah as children, their tiny fingers swishing the beads this way and that, counting and giggling at the rattling sound they made. I glance back at the door and wonder if they are OK on the other side of it.

As the morning wears on, the room fills up with other faces, all of them older than mine, a blankness and emptiness so apparent in their eyes, a faraway look already settling into their faces, filling the lines once made by laughter. Most of them are in couples, one wrinkly hand on top of another; some are with their children. I feel like I have been waiting a long time. I pick up the same magazine I had read a few weeks before, flicking through it again, cover to cover, reading the words, yet nothing going in.

I stare at the door, filling in the gaps of what might be happening beyond it. The neurologist will be assuring Sarah that I didn't want her to stay with me and be my carer, that actually it will be easier for me to live alone, that there will be less confusion, less chance of things being moved around.

Finally, there is a sound, a turn of the handle, thanks and goodbyes, the lightness of my girls' voices. I look up and scan their faces – no eyes red from tears – so the smile I greet them with is genuine, relieved. They smile their lovely smiles back at me, as if to say 'time to go home'. We leave the hospital, the mood much lighter as they chat about this and that, nothing of what had occurred behind closed doors. Maybe, like me, they need time for it to sink in too.

My strength returns in the cheeriness of their voices; it takes me immediately back to the roles I prefer, the ones we've honed so well over the years, when I am the mum who protects and shields them from all things bad. As we walk home, there are still things I can do to make life easier for them, to protect them in some small way. There will be a way of getting back some control. There's always a way.

Orange and lemon drizzle cakes were always the favourites. You knew the recipe off by heart: butter, flour, milk, sugar, eggs and lemon zest; you never needed to look it up. I remember the smell of your kitchen, the sweetness of a new sponge pulled fresh from the oven, the holes you'd stab into it, and the sticky lemon and orange syrup you'd drizzle into each one. The girls would stand waiting patiently, their eyes ready to eat, their noses touching the top of the kitchen worktop. 'It needs time to cool,' you'd tell them, and they'd go and play, running back downstairs when they heard the sound of the door, your friend arriving signalling the cutting of the first slice. You'd carefully carve pieces off it to put in their packed lunches; they always told you their friends were envious of their homemade cakes, which made you smile.

Every weekend or school holiday was an excuse for an afternoon of baking. You'd make miniature cupcakes – tiny buns for tiny hands – some iced with funny faces in different colours, Smarties for eyes and a red icing smile drawn with a steady grip. Some you'd top with marshmallows and edible pink glitter, or strawberry shoelaces snaked into an S for Sarah or a G for Gemma, and others topped with a mini cola bottle standing to attention, secured by a blob of icing. On other occasions, if time allowed, you'd lay out all the toppings and tiny squirty tubes of icing and the girls would create their own masterpieces, their faces full of concentration and pride at the final result.

You'd set them up outside in the garden on a sunny afternoon, Gemma on her plastic red chair that matched the miniature table, Sarah on a little wooden chair you'd painted yellow, and serve them afternoon tea on colourful paper plates you'd saved from parties. Less washing-up. They'd giggle as they tucked in and blobs of icing stuck to their noses.

A simple treat that made two little girls so happy, and all that love folded into the mixture.

The cookery book lies open on the worktop, well-thumbed pages speckled with stray ingredients. I quickly flick the page backwards and forwards and look into the bowl at the floury mixture that stares back. I lick a finger and dip it in – is that bicarbonate of soda? Or just flour? It's impossible to tell. I try to retrace my steps in the recipe, flick back and forth on the pages, back and forth, before fishing another teaspoon from the drawer and dropping another few grams into the mixture and watching the tiny light white cloud curl up in return.

In the last few months I've been baking cakes for a homeless charity in York. I'd seen an advert in the news-paper looking for volunteers for their breakfast service and I'd emailed to ask if a cake might be appreciated. I have always loved baking, but since my diagnosis there has been a shift in my mind; there's had to be. I've opened the wardrobe and seen the toes of my trainers lost under long hems at the back, and my car keys stayed in the red dish when I walked to the post office to send my driving licence back. So many compromises to make that I've wanted to – I've *needed* to – focus on what I still can do. Baking is something I can still do.

The first week I'd turned up, laden with Tupperware, the faces that gather at the shelter every Saturday morning eyed me and my two large Victoria sponges with suspicion.

'Why would you bake cakes for us?' one said.

'Everyone deserves a nice treat, don't they?' I replied. 'Anyway, I haven't got anyone else to bake for; you can be my critics.'

I never wanted them to think I felt sorry for them, I knew only too well how that felt. I like it at the shelter; no one knows me there, so they don't notice if a word abandons me mid-conversation, or if I forget someone's name from one week to the next. They don't know the old Wendy; they aren't watching me as closely as those who have worked with me for years, who are perplexed by the difference. I can relax there. I don't have to be on guard, disguising any slip-ups; these people are just grateful for my sweet offerings. I am known as the cake lady, a new identity I've carved from sugar and flour but one that suits me so much better than anything the doctors had written in my notes.

I turn back to my recipe and add in caster sugar.

The second week I'd arrived at the shelter, my arms full of chocolate cakes, I'd been presented with a dozen eggs by one of the homeless people, who'd spent his night sleeping in a barn.

'Now you've got no excuse not to come back next week.' He winked.

It feels nice to be useful, and I like the fact that they look forward to their cake on Saturday. I can't serve up a slice without thinking of my own girls and how, if they ever fell on hard times, I hope someone would do something nice for them. I realised, too, that the shelter's visitors didn't just need something for Saturday morning, they needed something to take away with them as well, so I started making rock cakes that would slip easily inside their pockets.

I flick back one page and forward again, I wrinkle my nose, then tip caster sugar into the bowl.

Some of them take being my critics very seriously indeed, giving me a detailed critique of my cake from one week to the next. Once a couple of new people turned up at the shelter and moaned that they didn't like what I'd baked that week, but the others had soon leapt to my defence. By then we'd built up a friendship.

I stop and scratch my head. Have I added caster sugar yet? I can't remember doing it. I look down into the bowl and see the granules so, relieved, I start mixing, but the spoon doesn't glide through the mixture like it usually does, it feels thicker, heavier. I tell myself I'll soon loosen it up, and work the spoon harder, which in turn makes my elbow ache. I pour the mixture into a loaf tin, but it clings to the side of the bowl instead of sliding off it. Odd, I think. I make a cup of tea while the cake is in the oven, but there's worry whittling away inside me. I keep casting a glance at the oven, getting up more than usual to peer through the glass door to see if it's rising.

At the shelter I often sit and have a cup of tea with the people who file in for something to eat on a Saturday morning. It is hard sometimes, listening to their stories, how their own families have deserted them and so in turn they have made family in each other. Being with them is grounding, however tough my week has been, however deep the pile of Post-it notes has grown on my carpet overnight, the meetings when I've felt suspicious eyes on me or heard the long sighs down the telephone receiver because I'm not grasping the problem quickly enough. And there's the fear I now wake and breathe and live with – the emptiness of what's to come. None of that exists at the shelter on Saturday mornings; there I'm reminded to be grateful for the things I still do have: a roof over my head, money to pay the bills, a shower and clean clothes to wear, two daughters who care so much.

Life can be cruel at times; it can steal so much in one hand that sometimes we just have to cling on to what it leaves behind, however small an offering. Sitting amongst these people whose world has deserted them often makes me think of all the plans you make when life is good. These people sitting around enjoying my cakes, taking care not to drop too many crumbs, must also have made plans like that during better moments in their lives. They too once had a home, a family, a job, yet here they are, relying on others for food and shelter, if only for a few hours. Given the hand that life had dealt them, they'd found tiny ways to make their lives better: the sleight of hand that pockets anything that can be saved for later, the compact way they stored their possessions, making it easier to carry their worldly goods from one door-way to another. They'd sought out help, giving support to one another. Often the older ones looked out for the younger ones, who might not have parents to fall back on. We all find ways of coping when we're ready to start searching for them.

I glance at the clock and it's time to get the loaf out of the oven, but in the kitchen there's a strange smell, something different. I pull it carefully from the shelf and pat it with my oven gloves; it hasn't risen and it looks hard and stodgy. I turn it out on a cooling tray, but it doesn't look right and I can't work out why. I wait twenty minutes, and then slice off the end, but the knife sticks through it, the sponge doesn't spring back happily as it usually does; inside it's dense and compacted, a heaviness where air usually is. I try a corner but wrinkle up my face. It's inedible. Too sweet, too much sugar. It goes straight into the bin. I look at the other Tupperware neatly stacked on my worktop and realise with a sinking feeling that there's not enough, that someone will have to go without this week.

I stare at the cake in the bin. It isn't the first time this has happened. The rock cakes had too much salt last week. Another Victoria sponge had gone in the bin the week before. I know why. It's because I can't follow the recipe. I used to store it all in my head and now I follow it from the book, but I turn the page and *poof*, it's gone. Last week I mixed up teaspoons and tablespoons. The week before it had been double flour. Sadness wells inside and with it a frustration and anger that has been building for weeks. I look at the cake, broken and useless inside the bin. I have heard nothing from any doctor since my diagnosis three months ago, nothing but one appointment at the memory clinic, and that is still weeks away. How can I help my daughters understand my diagnosis if I can't understand it myself? That's what I feel angry about. That's why I feel broken and abandoned, discarded by an NHS that I have worked in for twenty years. Surely I, more than anyone, know how the system works. I am the system; I manage the system. And yet the system has abandoned me.

I close the bin. I don't want to look at that cake any more. I know I won't go back to the shelter. I don't want to explain why I keep getting it wrong; better to slip off radar, however much the guilt and sadness sting. I feel empty inside. Yes, the emptiness for the insights I'll no longer be privy to at the shelter, the way I've found the people who visit there so inspiring, but more than anything, a real, visceral grief at saying another goodbye, this time to baking, something I've done my whole life. From baking the first fairy cakes as a child to teaching my girls how to do the same, it's always been there, a constant. There wasn't a gloomy day that a bit of baking couldn't cheer. I stare at the long line of cookery books in the kitchen, those with pages that are wrinkled and bent, others clean and bright, and yet I know now I'll never get round to using them. Another goodbye, this time to something so sweet. But I think of those people at the shelter, how the things they've lost would make mine pale by comparison. And yet they found a way to make life that bit easier by seeking out help.

I go to my filing cabinet and pull out all the medical letters I can find, all the correspondence that has dropped into my hand or through my letterbox since my diagnosis. I find the names and telephone numbers of those who should have contacted me and of those organisations that might be able to unravel this mystery inside my brain. I rattle off emails asking for, even demanding help. Not just for me, but so I can help my daughters. I need to understand what Alzheimer's is and what it means for me.

It's Saturday morning and three blank documents sit staring at me from the yellow-and-white-checked tablecloth. I see some pencil marks I've made on my copy, and feel my fingers twist the tea towel in my hands. This is going to be hard. I turn my attention instead back to the kitchen worktop, the tiny buns I've recently pulled from the oven, and take deep, sweet breaths of the scent that fills that room. It's almost all ready: miniature lemon drizzle cakes, teeny Victoria sponges, each one a favourite of the girls. There are tiny sandwiches too, and very carefully I cut the crusts off each one, and lay them beside the mini quiches. I then search the back of my cupboards for some edible glitter, sprinkling some on each perfect little cake before arranging them on the cake stand. The documents watch me from the table, and I swallow down the pain that I'm trying to disguise with shimmering dust. I spy the glass cabinet, and inside my white and gold-rimmed tea service adorned with pretty pink roses and daisies. I lay the table, three cups on three saucers, matching plates and milk jug. I even fill a bowl with sugar cubes, placing the silver tongs on top, despite the fact that none of us even take sugar in our tea.

I stand back and look at the table, very proud of my efforts and the way the tea has turned out. But I also know that we may not be in the mood to eat any of it, that all of this may have been for nothing, although it's the only way I have of sweetening this bitter moment. Today Gemma and Sarah are on their way round to help me write my lasting power of attorney document – in effect, what my wishes are when I'm no longer able to articulate them. I think of some of the questions that I've already written in pencil, and fight that feeling inside that so desperately wants to protect my girls from having to do this.

A moment later, I hear the sound of car doors outside, the click of the garden gate signalling their arrival.

'Mmmm, something smells good,' Sarah says as they come through the door. Amidst the hugs and kisses, I see them glance at the paperwork waiting on the table.

'Let's get the boring bit out of the way, then we can get on with the serious business of afternoon tea,' I say, trying to lighten their nervousness. Or is that mine?

I suggest we start with the section on finance. It's fairly straightforward and I'm glad of the pencil comments I've already made and the silence it fills explaining them. We move on to the health section next. Their heads are bowed now. I spot the glances to one another for reassurance every so often. I clear my throat.

'Question six – restrictions about health and welfare,' I say. Noticing the subtle but sharp intake of breath from both, I put the paperwork down. 'I don't want to be resuscitated.'

There is a moment's silence. 'I can understand that,' Gemma says.

Sarah is silent. I can see the aspiring nurse is struggling, that she knows this goes against everything she is training for, that life must be fought for. But not mine. Not this life.

'What are you thinking, Sarah?'

There's a pause. 'But what if you might pull through?' she says. 'What if you just required antibiotics to recover?'

I sense the desperation in her voice and for a second I'm blindsided. I shouldn't be here, shouldn't be explaining to my girls why I wouldn't want to stay in the world with them.

'But if Mum had already lost capacity and we were making those decisions for her, she wouldn't want to survive and continue to deteriorate with dementia in control,' Gemma says gently. 'She wouldn't want to get better and live in the dementia world.'

I smile, feeling the breath I've been holding on to leave me.

'Good job we're talking now, otherwise you'd be falling out and arguing over decisions when I couldn't help put things right,' I say with a smile, trying in some way to brighten the mood.

Sarah nods, an internal reminder that we're here to talk about my wishes. It's done. That emotional decision filed away, done and dusted until a time when it's needed. A time I hope will be a long way in the future, but who knows?

I turn back to the document, my finger scans down the page, and a knot pulls tight inside my stomach, indicating where I need to stop.

'I'm sure we've spoken of this before, but this is what I've written in pencil: "If I no longer have the mental capacity to choose my place of residence or become unsafe at home, my attorneys have my approval to choose a suitable residential home …"' I pause. Both of them are looking at their laps. 'I never want you to be my carers. You're my daughters and always will be.'

'Yes, we know, Mum,' Sarah says softly. 'If you're sure …'

I pick up a pen and go over the words in ink, but even as I do, something doesn't feel right, because I know this isn't what I want, to end up in a home, but it'll have to do for now. It's better than the thought of my girls giving up their lives to care for me.

Even the room seems to sigh with relief once it's over, everything signed and dated, boxes ticked, the final legalities read out. The three of us sit there for a while, a time that feels like minutes, but is perhaps only seconds, the red clock on the wall keeping pace with our thoughts.

I break the silence. 'Let's open the door – it's become very warm in here. And who's going to help me lay out tea?'

With that the papers are put to one side and we turn our attention to the cakes.

'Aw, look how tiny they are,' Gemma says.

I pour the tea and we take tiny bites of lemon drizzle sponge, the sugar sweetening the rest of the afternoon, just like it was meant to.

The upturned box of photographs is scattered across the ivory lace duvet. I pick one from the pile and turn it over in my hands; Sarah and Gemma, aged around six and three, chubby legs neatly fitted inside towelling shorts on a sandy beach. I smile as the moment comes back to me: our first holiday just the three of us, I-spy games on the journey and counting different coloured cars, favourite sweets to make the time go faster, brand-new boxes of wax crayons and bumper colouring books opened on the way. We'd arrived at our chalet on the Norfolk coast, dumped our bags and run straight to the sea, and this photograph was taken the first moment their feet sank into the sand. I could still hear their excited squeals as a far-too-cold sea ran up and tickled between their toes.

Then something else washes over me, a sadness that has been growing inside me for weeks. Am I really going to forget all this? Will I, one day soon, clutch this photograph in my hands and not know the two happy faces that smile back? It doesn't seem possible. I feel an urgency, staring hard at the photograph, determined to outwit my fading brain, to memorise every pixel of it; a big blue

Norfolk sky, the pink flip-flops in Sarah's hands I hadn't noticed before, Gemma's navy-and-red-striped shorts, other holidaymakers on the beach. A photograph where once I only saw the girls is now suddenly filled with tiny details. I will store it to memory. I won't let it slip away. I turn the photograph over and write on the back: *Sarah and Gemma. Norfolk holiday. Caister? 1987.*

I won't forget.

I pick another photograph from the pile, me sitting on top of Walla Crag in Keswick. It's a moody day, the sun squeezing through just one or two gaps in the low-slung clouds, the darkness of Derwentwater below, and me looking out at the view laid before me – beautiful despite the weather – a striped Breton top and my red rucksack cutting through the gloom of the day. I shuffle to the edge of my bed and feel the springs relent. I clutch the photograph between two fingers and I stare at the view again, burning it to memory, telling myself that from here, in my cream and olive bedroom, I can still pretend I am there, feeling the whoosh of the wind in my ears, smelling the damp moss beneath my feet, hearing the emptiness of the silence. It's all there, the memories that I now long to hold fast to, they haven't left me yet. I can still conjure up the feelings that go hand in hand with them, the peace that the beauty of the place brings, the warmth wrapped inside my coat on a breezy day. Those are the feelings I need to clutch more tightly; the calm, the happiness. I'm determined that even when I can't name the place, the feelings won't desert me.

I look around my spare room and feel a sudden desire to pin these photographs all over the blank walls, to create a space that I can wander into whenever the fog descends. I brush my hands through the pile of photographs, all the very best moments of my life captured on film, and I'm grateful for every time my finger pressed down on the shutter. I had no idea then just how much I would come to rely on these photographs, that I would develop a disease that would steal memories from me, that every day something more cherished than any of my possessions would be lost. That's what Alzheimer's does: it's a thief in the night, stealing precious pictures from our lives while we sleep.

I start from the beginning then, sifting through the photographs and quickly scribbling down whatever detail I can muster; names and places and dates, an insurance policy against memory loss. I write quickly, making the most of today's active brain, reaching from one photograph to another, my arms aching, my mind tiring, but not daring to stop in case the momentum is lost. With each one I stare harder, fixing every detail deeper inside, alert for clues I may have missed before, my life whizzing past as the pile gets smaller.

There is one photograph left, a view of the river from one of my favourite bridges in York. I scan every wave the water makes and find within it a whirlpool I've never noticed before, a clue to the life that dwells beneath the water's surface, a tiny detail I'd missed when I'd been taking in the bigger picture with my lens. I make a mental note to search for it next time I pass the same spot on the bridge. Then I decide to swap a mental note for a written one. Just to be safe.

The following day I'm wandering through York, the note crumpled inside my pocket. I go to the bridge and stand looking out at the same view that I'd captured in the photograph, and there it is, as promised, the water swirling just as I knew it would be, just how it had been in the photograph. I stand on the bridge staring down, a sense of achievement I can't quite name bubbling beneath the surface. I know it is inevitable that dementia will steal these memories from me, that in the future I might not recognise the whirlpool in the picture, or the bridge, or even the town where the photo was taken, yet I am happy to know that nature will ensure these things survive, that the whirlpool keeps on whirling, that the sea keeps on lapping on sandy shores where we had holidays filled with love and laughter. Dementia won't steal everything, even though it can feel that way now. Even though forgetting my daughters is my worst fear, nature will ensure that the tides rise, the sun sets, the brooks keep on babbling. I am heartened to understand that dementia is nothing more than a trick of my mind, and I can outwit it if I stare at my photographs hard enough, if I find the whirlpool that is still there – the tiny gem to be appreciated in all this.

That day in York I buy all I need to create my memory room and I go home and string up dozens of photographs across the walls, securing each one with a brightly coloured miniature peg. I flick every one over as I do, and there they are, the prompts that I scribbled down yesterday – the whys, the whos, the wheres – there to help me for a time when I won't remember.

I finish and stand back to look at my work; colourful photos of Sarah and Gemma from all different times in their childhood stare back from one line, on another all the houses I've ever lived in, another is filled with photographs of some of my favourite views – the Lake District, the Dorset coast, Blackpool beach. I sit on the edge of the bed in front of them, feeling that same sense of calm and happiness. When the memories have emptied on the inside, they'll still be here on the outside – a constant, a reminder, a feeling of happier times. Will it be next week, next month, next year? I don't know. That thought alone stirs a fear inside, an urgency to remember everything while I still have the chance, but I calm the panic by focusing on one picture, the view from Walla Crag. I'm up there again, the wind whistling in my ears, the damp moss beneath my feet. The uncertain future can wait.

I know life wasn't easy for you, I didn't always acknowledge that at the time. There was always so much to do, so much to think about, lists to write, mouths to feed. There wasn't always time to just sit and reflect in front of a steaming cup of tea. How many single mums ever remember to give themselves a pat on the back?

The girls' dad left when they were just seven and four. I know it was tough. I know life was lonely. I know you worked hard to hide these things from the girls, painting a smile on your face and being determined not to let it slip. I remember that even if you did a good job of hiding it from others by making a joke, too proud to let it slip, and never in front of the girls, life was difficult.

There wasn't much money to go round, so you always had to be organised. Getting ready for Christmas often meant selling little bits and bobs before you could find more to fill their stockings with. You didn't feel hard done by or want pity; instead you enjoyed the challenge. There was the second-hand bike that you sanded down and repainted ready for Sarah's excited squeals on 25 December. And the farmyard playset you made yourself while the girls slept, complete with a tinfoil pond stuck to the cardboard with love. Every year you stayed up on Christmas Eve long after the girls sank into dreams of Santa, and wrote out the 'Christmas Menu' for the next day — right down to games you'd all play, the turkey and all the trimmings. Gemma and Sarah say now they never remember going without, but it took a lot of doing.

You had to be creative with days out too. Most often it was a trip to the library for story time, where books were free and the rooms were warm. The girls, too, could escape to a far-off land of make-believe.

I always got the sense you rather liked not having much money. It made life a challenge, made you have to think harder, be more organised. Two of the things you love the most. Which seems ironic now.

There was nothing in life you couldn't fix with a Mr Men book, you'd say. Whenever the girls had a problem you'd fish out the right one. Gemma was always so shy, so you'd read Little Miss Shy until the pages were worn with thumbprints, and the story bedded deep into her mind. When Sarah was worrying, out came Mr Worry. The world always looked a tad less scary afterwards. If only there had been a Mr Men book for you in those days.

The hardest moments for you were letting them go to stay with their dad at weekends and holidays. Never a cross word or criticism raised — after all, he was their dad. But how the house *seemed so empty and quiet when they'd gone, your heart ripped out and packed off in the suitcase with them. It was when they weren't there that the worry hit hardest; you'd never been able to have a proper job after he left, as any work had to fit in with school. You'd slotted in as many cleaning jobs as you could, often recommended by word of mouth, which at least made it more bearable. But you knew you were worth more. Those jobs had served their purpose while the girls were tiny, but now they were getting older, both of them at school, there had to be something else out there.*

In those dark days you learned the art of distancing yourself from the problem by floating up and looking down on yourself, and asking if there was another way. I try to do the same now, but the answers aren't coming like they did back then ...

I shuffle into my bedroom, sleep rattling inside, my head craving a soft pillow. I glance at the novel patiently waiting on my bedside table and quickly look away. It's a reminder of how I might have once spent the last waking hours and minutes. Another evening, I tell myself, knowing the folded page hasn't shifted in weeks. But my eyes fall on something else beside it – a Post-it note: *Book dentist appointment.* I sigh and roll my eyes, was it any surprise that I had forgotten all about it? Even the little notes I've been leaving myself for months are starting to fail me now – what good is a note to yourself if you forget to look for it? A scribble made in the night, or even the morning, is now often forgotten about by lunchtime, more often by the time I leave the house. I prop the note up next to the clock, determined tomorrow that I will remember to call the dental surgery.

The following morning, I wake to a selection of other notes, I scoop them from the floor, flicking through them as I make my first cup of Yorkshire tea. As I do, I notice the pillbox by the kettle, yesterday's tablets still sitting inside. Even remembering to take my medication is becoming a challenge, and the notes scrunched up inside my hand prove that they are not reminder enough. I sit down with my tea and pick up my iPad. Perhaps the answer is on here. I see an icon that says 'reminder' and type in *7 p.m., take tablets*. It's worth a try.

I arrive home from work exhausted that evening, but when I hear the buzzer on my iPad I open it up. *Take tablets*, it says. I wander into the kitchen and swallow down the tablets with a glass of water. And it gets me thinking. I pull the calendar down from the wall and start to fill my iPad with important dates, times and reminders – doctor's appointments, friends' visits, a daily reminder to take my tablets, to put the rubbish bins out. I hesitate over 17 October, Sarah's birthday, just a few weeks away. Surely I would never forget a date as important as that, but just in case I set a reminder for the evening of her birthday.

As the day approaches, an alarm goes off on my iPad to remember to buy Sarah a card. I smile to myself and glance across at the kitchen worktop where the card lies waiting to be written in. A couple of days later, another reminder, this time to post it, but I see it already has the name and address written on it, a stamp duly in place in the top right-hand corner. I settle back with my cup of tea, a warm feeling inside with each sip, a happiness that my instincts had been right, that I hadn't forgotten Sarah's birthday, that love could and would outwit dementia every time. But then something inside goes cold, a worry starts to whittle away. I feel my eyebrows knit together into a question mark: would the card have been waiting to be posted if I hadn't set the first alarm? But I remind myself that I never forget a birthday, it's one of my things. I post the card that morning, while I remember.

On 17 October I go to work like any other day, and I come home and set about making myself something to eat. I'm humming along to a tune on the radio when I hear a ping from my iPad. I glance up at the clock: 6.30 p.m., so not quite time for my tablets. Puzzled, I put down the utensils I'd been using and open up the iPad to see *Sarah's birthday* as the reminder. My insides turn icy cold. It can't be. There must be a mistake. I must have done something wrong. I would have always called her in the morning to wish her a happy birthday. I check the date on the calendar, abandon my meal and reach for the phone. I'm shaking as I dial Sarah's number, as I hear the ringtone, her voice answering.

'I'm so sorry,' I say. 'I-I don't know how it happened.'

'It's OK,' she says. 'You just forgot.' I can sense from the warmth in her voice that she means it, that she understands, that she's smiling, but that icy coldness in my stomach doesn't let go, it clings on tighter, even when she tells me she got my card, even when I hang up the phone. Nothing can ease the sadness, the mortification: I've forgotten my own daughter's birthday for the first time in thirty-four years. A day that means more to me than almost 364 others. My logical mind knows that it's the disease, not me, but on a day like today it's hard to tell us apart. For the first time I really hate dementia, for what it's stolen, for what it's about to steal. I can't forgive it, or myself.

A mind can't help fast forwarding, willing a happy event to hurry towards us, or agonising over that very same future in a darker light. There aren't many of us who are content enough to live in the here and now. Instead we go about our daily lives thinking we have all the time in the world to worry and whittle about the minor distractions in our day: the grumpy colleague, a bus running late, the rain breaking through the clouds when we've forgotten an umbrella. How many times do we sit there on a Monday at work and wish the weekend would come? Or hope the weeks would fly past for a long-awaited holiday? And then something comes along that stops us right in our tracks — a divorce, a death, a progressive illness. Something that reminds us there is only today.

That feeling — the need to remember everything, to burn things on to my mind like film before it's too late — has been creeping towards me each day since my diagnosis, and is what powered me to create a memory room. I'll be sitting at my desk and feel that urgency pushing towards me like a wave. Everything I know about my job — all that information I have stored inside my mental filing cabinets, the same ones my colleagues are used to accessing in a second — rushes forwards, and I fear the moment when that same wave crashes, scattering that information across the sand before the tide sweeps it back into a vast ocean, that individual wave and everything within it lost for ever.

I scan all the folders on my desktop and feel panic inside. Over the last five years I have gathered all the information to ensure the roster system runs without fault, but much of it is now stored inside my mind, not in these virtual envelopes. With my memory becoming increasingly unreliable, how will I even know when this information is lost? Could it be next week? Next month? Tomorrow? I've noticed in recent days that my staff look up at me, confused, when I've shown them around the desktop of my computer, or offered to run them through the finer workings of the roster.

'You know that sister can't do nights,' I tell them. 'She has young children. You should make a note of that somewhere.'

But I can see what they're thinking: *Why do we need to when we have you?* There's one particular member of staff who I have earmarked as the next 'guru', the one who will be well placed to take my title, and I find myself calling her in for meetings more frequently, sharing my workload with her, showing her more and more details about my role while I still can. She's as capable as I knew she would be, diligently taking notes, but in my mind they're never fast enough, there's not enough paper in her pad or ink in her pen, there isn't enough time to get everything out that is necessary, everything they'll need once I'm gone. Or at least on the days that cloud over, when horizons become blurred.

I sit on the bus home, looking out for landmarks in a bid to beat sleep from settling on my shoulders. What will tomorrow bring? A clear day or a foggy one? And what's the forecast? Will this disease's descent on me be a temperate one for the week ahead? I tell myself not to think further than today, but it's impossible, especially when I'm tired, too fatigued to keep the fear at bay. It's always the same three things that whittle away inside, and each time the thought of one creeps in, the other two leap to join it. The fear of losing my independence, of being unable to get a bus to and from town, let alone work. I glance at my ghostly reflection in the bus window, a reminder of another major fear: going over the edge into someone I don't recognise, losing a grip on what makes me *me*. A time when decisions will be made for me, not by me. And then that naturally leads to the third fear, so painful that each time it comes to me I feel my heart twist in response: forgetting the faces of the two people who are most dear to me, Sarah and Gemma. My heart races then, out of control just like my thoughts, just like my future. Are these fears that we all face? Of losing independence and, eventually, our faculties? Fears that always seemed so far away, tiny dots on the horizon that once I would have had to squint to see. But dementia has sent me hurtling towards them. No wonder there is that sense of urgency, to fit in a future before it disappears forever. Will it be a slow goodbye or a quick one? The uncertainty is what fills my chest with panic. The not knowing how quickly time will become irrelevant. I thought I had life under control. Hadn't I pictured retirement a long way from now, my car and me, driving to all the places in the British Isles too far to reach within a week's annual leave? Hadn't I just started earning enough to plan trips further afield, long weekends in Dublin, Paris? Wasn't I going to see the world? What happened to all that time I thought I had?

How much time do you think you lost scouring the small ads in the local newspaper? Your finger ran down the page from job to job, week in, week out, searching for that perfect position until the tip of it was black with ink. You knew you could be more than a cleaner, that there could be more for you than scrubbing sinks and toilets while the girls were at school, but finding something to fit in with the family rhythm was the hardest. You did it for five years after their dad left, just to get by, but you knew there had to be more to life than that.

And then one day you saw the perfect job: part-time receptionist in the physiotherapy department at Milton Keynes Hospital. The advert promised flexibility: you could work mornings or afternoons. That active mind of yours that I so envy now started to race with the possibilities, persuading yourself that the girls would appreciate a bit of responsibility and independence, either getting themselves to school or home. Sarah was old enough by then to look after them both if you were a little later than the school bell. You were full of hope as you called for an application form, smiling down the receiver, finding it impossible to keep the excitement from your voice.

When the paperwork arrived a few days later, you sat at the kitchen table and stared at the blanks you were supposed to fill in. Current Employment *gave you a bit of pause, but you did what you always did and tackled the issue head on.*

'Cleaner' would hardly impress them you feared, but there was no hiding it: You may wonder why someone who is now a cleaner thinks she may be suitable for the advertised post of receptionist ... *you wrote, and then proceeded to give them all the reasons why you were an excellent candidate for the job: your memory and attention to detail, to name just two, and the fact that you were quick to learn. So different from now. But they wrote back and you got an interview, and years later, long after they'd given you the job and you'd moved up and through the ranks, one of the people who interviewed you explained how she'd persuaded the other manager to give you a chance, that being a single mum of two gave you more reason than many to work hard and hang on to your job. And that's just what you did. You were thirty-nine and someone had thrown you a life-line. That job was the start of a twenty-year career in the NHS, where you'd become so devoted to your job you were accused of being a workaholic, that when you had a stroke it was the stress of the job, the hours you put in, that were to blame. But for the first time in your life you had real independence, and you were so determined to hang on to it.*

The table is in a long narrow room and I sit at the end, waiting for the rest of the seats to fill up. I'm excited, a smile stuck fast to my face, and with a sense of something I haven't felt in a while: the ability to contribute and change minds. I'd found out about the Dementia Friends initiative on the Alzheimer's Society website, and I'd become a friend by watching the video explaining life with the disease – as if I needed telling – but at the end there was more: a chance to spread the word further than the internet by becoming what they called a Dementia Friends Champion. That is the training I'm here for now. I thought of my friends and colleagues at work, and enrolled on this local course. Silently others file into the room, and we start by introducing ourselves.

'I work at St James's Hospital in Leeds; I was diagnosed with dementia in July and I need a simple way to explain to my team and make others aware of dementia,' I tell them. 'I think if a person with dementia delivers a session it would have a bigger impact.'

There is silence from every seat at the table, all eyes on me. It's obvious in that long second that I am the only person in the room who actually has dementia, and, ironically, even though the others came to learn how to share more about the disease, they hadn't expected to be sitting alongside someone who has it. It feels like an age before the next person speaks.

'Thank you for sharing, Wendy,' the facilitator says finally. 'Right, who's next?'

She moves on. Each person has their own reason for being here today, and then we listen and learn as she presents different tools and ways that we can help people to understand dementia. During the break for lunch people come over one by one to tell me how much they admire my reason for being here, but I see that just my presence alone is breaking one myth about the disease for all of us – reminding us that it isn't age-related.

We learn lots of different techniques for sharing information, including a fun game of bingo where the facilitator reads out helpful sound bites about dementia and we have to find the missing words on our bingo cards. By the afternoon, I feel my own nerves starting to bite inside; it's almost my turn to deliver part of the Dementia Friends session to the room. I'm shaking inside as I walk up to the front, despite the fact that I have written down a speech during my lunch hour, underlining key words that I mustn't forget. I take a deep breath and start talking, I hold the attention of the room, growing in confidence as I do, thinking how all those years of training skills at work must be holding me in good stead, that they're still in there somewhere.

'Before we start, maybe I should dispel another myth. So many people, when they hear the word "dementia", think of the end. Maybe some of you thought that too. Well, I'm here before you to show how dementia has a beginning before the end and so much life to live in between. Don't give up on us, as no matter what stage we're at, we still have so much to give. We just might give in different ways.'

I see them relax in their seats, understanding more now than when they arrived this morning. I get through it, and the room applauds.

At the end of the session, many of the others come up to me.

'I just don't feel so wary about dementia now,' one says.

'I'm no longer uncertain about how to talk to someone with the disease,' another says.

I leave the room, like all the others, a Dementia Champion. I'm still coming to terms with the disease myself, but at least I know how to tell people what it means to have Alzheimer's. Just as soon as I'm ready.

The last Post-It note is crumpled inside my hand and I manage to get it into the bin under my desk in time to hear the first of my colleagues arriving at the office. I have been here an hour already, and my wastepaper basket is already filled with notes I've been working through in preparation for the day ahead.

'Morning,' I call to my colleague, my head under the desk, ensuring none of the paper is visible, that no one can see just what I need to do to keep my job. I come back up for air, my guilty secret of six months tucked away somewhere near my feet. More and more recently it has felt like I am leading a double life. There's the person I project to those around me, trying to emulate the one they're more used to, and the new me, the one who is so determined to hide mistakes or the extra time it takes to get through basic tasks.

While the rest of the office has been embracing tutorials in a new roster system, the multicoloured squares it uses to organise and categorise have remained a mystery to me, despite all the extra hours I've put in at home after work, or before work when the office is quiet and I have nothing but the hum of the photocopier for company. It just hasn't clicked for me; it remains mysterious. The implementation of the system is only weeks away, so I know I can't hide my confusion with it much longer. The worst thing is that they are going to see it soon too, and then I will fall from office guru to the idiot who can't keep up. Day by day, I am losing control, and the frustration is biting inside. Dementia hasn't yet stolen all the knowledge I still have on the art of rostering, even if I can't keep up with the new system. I'm not yet completely redundant. But I am keeping a secret, and sometimes the guilt of that stings.

I have been hoping to carry on working for as long as possible, but hiding my diagnosis is becoming harder every day. In fact, it's becoming more exhausting than the job itself. I am constantly looking out for clues that will jog my fading memory as to who is on the other end of the phone; finding it difficult to concentrate in the office with all the noise of phones and conversations;

wasting time going over and over the same task that previously would have taken me seconds to complete. I wonder if anyone notices how many times I leave my phone unanswered. Or maybe it's just me who knows the art of multitasking has deserted me. But I'm afraid to tell people, that's the truth of it.

As the office fills up with smiling faces, I look around and realise I don't want my staff to look at me with pity rather than respect or my managers to question my capability. But in truth, how much longer can I keep up this facade? I know I need to tell them before the dementia takes the decision out of my hands and makes itself known directly. Anyway, I reason – as I have reasoned a dozen times before when the same thought has occurred – I work in a hospital, surely that should give me the confidence to ask for advice and support to keep on working, especially if we're striving all the time to provide a dementia-friendly place for patients.

I turn back to my screen and open a new email. I write the names of my three managers at the top and start to type. It wasn't going to be an easy conversation for any of us, so I decide to tell them about my diagnosis by email first; that way they have time to digest and discuss it between them before they speak to me. I write openly but practically, explaining clearly what I'm still capable of, what I find difficult and how I think I might find it easier, knowing they want solutions, not problems. And then I press send. I listen to the muted chatter of my own staff in adjacent offices, but of course none of them have noticed a thing. Next, I schedule appointments with each manager in turn over the next few days, and then I sit back in my chair, anxious and relieved to have shared the news, to have reached out for support, and just hoping it won't change everything. I leave for the day, just in case any of them surprise me by ringing there and then or popping their heads around the door. Unlikely, but best not to leave it to chance.

Two days later I knock on my immediate manager's door for the first meeting. My heart is beating so hard I wonder if it can be seen through my shirt. I tell myself he doesn't know how nervous I am; in fact, he seems more hesitant than me as I walk in and sit down in front of him.

'I'll admit I don't have much knowledge of dementia ...' he begins.

I try to explain the little that I know, what I first noticed, the difficulties I have at work.

'How long have you got?' he asks.

This time it was the question, not the dementia that stole the words from me. I pause for a second, trying to put myself in his shoes, to take the sting out of the words. I know exactly what he wants me to tell him: how long before I'm useless at work. I'd gone in prepared, knowing questions a little like these might be raised, hoping they wouldn't.

'Maybe you should refer me to occupational health?' I suggest calmly, taking the lead because I can see he is struggling. 'I'm not ready to retire. I've been diagnosed with dementia, but that doesn't mean that I've suddenly lost my ability to work, I just need to adapt a little so I can carry on working; they'll know how to facilitate that.'

I suggest working from home every other day. That way I'll have the quiet I need to be able to concentrate. He agrees, but as I leave his office he seems unconvinced. Everything I feared has come true: the pity *is* unavoidable. I see it in his eyes as I close his door behind me.

Another knock at another door. It is a month later and this is my first meeting with the occupational health consultant. I'm not nervous, as I was when meeting with my manager, as cases like mine are this doctor's job. She will have considered things I haven't, and make suggestions that will help me feel more empowered and more able to work for longer. I have been working every other day from home for the last four weeks and it has helped a little. I am still slower, but much more able to concentrate. My own staff have just assumed I need more time to recover after the stroke. I let them think that, not ready to reveal my new diagnosis to them. Certainly not until I've had the chance to speak to occupational health and know just what will be put into place to help me to continue working.

I push open the door and as I do, the doctor spins round to greet me, but my eyes fall not on her smile or the pitying tilt of her head, but on the computer behind her, a webpage I recognise, a regular now on my list of favourites at home. She has been looking at the website for the Alzheimer's Society, and the heading on the page reads: *Symptoms of Dementia*. She glances behind her and sees what I've spotted.

'Oh ... I ...' She closes the screen quickly, turns her computer away slightly just to be doubly sure. 'I've found a great website and there's lots of information ...'

'Yes,' I say. 'I know that page well.'

'Yes, of course.'

She looks embarrassed as I sit down with my file of paperwork, and I'm trying hard to ignore the sinking feeling inside, the thought that says I've already equipped myself with more knowledge than any of these so-called professionals.

Just like my manager, she tells me that she's never been involved in advising someone on living well with dementia.

'Never mind *working* well,' she says with an awkward smile.

She starts flicking through paperwork and I glance through it as she does from my side of the desk. There's nothing about the adaptations required for work; it's all about ill-health retirement, NHS pensions. I want to scream that I'm not ready, but instead I sit quietly and bite my tongue until I can't resist any longer.

'I am still managing my team efficiently. I just have some trouble getting to grips with the new——'

'Have you considered ill-health retirement? I can help with all the forms you need,' she says, looking through my file.

The notes I'd made sit abandoned inside my folders. It is as if the decision had already been made for me before I even entered the room. I watch as she makes notes and fills in forms, her pen skipping along, ticking boxes. She doesn't look up to include me. Perhaps she thinks she's making it easier for me this way, making the decisions so I don't have to. Others have also suggested I retire due to sickness, but I've shunned the idea. I'm not sick – I am well; I just need help and advice. But it's sadness, not anger that wells inside me.

She has a form in front of her where she needs to write her recommendations, and I sit watching, helpless as she begins to fill in one particular section: *Incapable of meeting the demands of her NHS employment* …

My fate has been decided.

I still have a mortgage to pay, so reducing my hours was never an option. I won't be able to pay the bills, and so, just as she's suggested, early retirement is the best way. At least then I'll get a lump sum to pay off my mortgage. I'm trying so hard to look at the positives. But as I leave her office, clutching a copy of the form she filled in, any hope I had in the health system evaporates. The system itself, my manager, even occupational health — they've all abandoned me. I have been able to advise them far more than they have me. I am working within the NHS and I still can't get the support I need. What chance do others with dementia have? I know I still have a valuable contribution to make and I'm not ready to write myself off. I have worked hard to get to where I am and I don't feel ready to give it all up. It seems like I'm shouting and screaming into the wind. I am not sick. I want to be heard. I am angry, but more than anything, I am sad and deflated.

I'm back at my desk, trying to shrug off the hopeless feeling I've had since the meetings with my managers and occupational health. The office starts to fill with the sounds of my team arriving; calls of 'good morning' fill my ears and that warmth returns, a trust deep inside replacing the unknowns.

I know I've got to tell them. They'll be shocked, but I know they'll help me. For the last few weeks I've been mulling over just how to break it to them; an email doesn't seem personal enough, but blurting it out in a meeting seems too direct. I know they're worth more than that. My team is made up of lots of different characters, each with their own unique set of skills. There are those who offer a quiet, steady hand, not saying much, just getting the job done, adapting as required, and there are the ones who will ask questions, determined to deepen their understanding and give more. Both sets of people are, and will be, much needed in the coming ... weeks? Months? Who knows?

I look up at my screen. It has gone to sleep, and two words run across it in bright colourful letters: *Dementia Awareness*. I stare and watch as they cross the screen, and again. There are often initiatives brought in at work, little messages sent to our screens by IT at the request of managers much higher up in the hospital who want us to focus on a particular corner of learning. This month, coincidentally, it's dementia. It comes to me: the bingo cards and other fun techniques I learned a few weeks ago at the Dementia Friends session. I smile to myself. This is how I'll do it.

A week later I'm standing in a meeting room with eight faces staring back at me – half of my team, who I've carefully selected. The other half is back in the office, waiting for their training session later in the day. They've no idea why they're here, although I've heard the whispers around the office; most just assume it's part of the hospital drive to learn more about dealing with patients with dementia. The room is smaller than I'd hoped, the windows shut, and as I look out at my staff from the front of the room, it suddenly feels hot, claustrophobic, eight bodies squeezed into a room meant for four.

'Can someone open a window at the back?' I ask, raising my voice above their gentle mutters. And then I begin. 'You may have noticed the "Dementia Awareness" icon criss-crossing your screen over the last few days ...'

A few heads go down, there are some awkward shuffles. Some hadn't noticed at all. That's OK.

'Well, today I thought I'd take you through a Dementia Friends session.'

On the table in front of them are bingo cards. They have different words written on them: *Alzheimer's, progressive, living well, short-term memory*. I've deliberately started with a fun game, me reading out sentences with key words missing, them ticking off the ones on their card they think are relevant. As we get going, the mood lightens, someone calls out 'Bingo' when they get a line, and I hand out a chocolate. There are smiles, laughter even; this is just how I wanted it to be. We carry on to see who can complete the whole card first.

'Dementia is not a natural part of ...' I say, leaving them to fill in the rest of the sentence.

'Bingo!' they all shout in unison, and we all laugh then. I hand out the last of the chocolates and pick up the notes in front of me, noticing as I do my hands are shaking ever so slightly. I start to read.

'You might like to think of the memory of someone with dementia as a bit like a bookcase as tall as I am. A cheap, mass-produced, flat-pack bookcase. This bookcase is full of books that contain factual memories. The top shelf – the ones you have to stand on your tiptoes to reach – hold very recent memories, such as what you had for breakfast this morning. By your shoulders are books from perhaps your fifties, the ones that all of us are used to reaching out and taking from the shelf any time we like – no effort, hardly any strain. And by your knees are books from your twenties. And then you get all the way down to your feet, where just beyond the tips of your toes you'll find books from your childhood. Having dementia rocks your bookcase from side to side, and it's always the books at the top that fall first, jumbling everything else up, so sometimes what you think of as your most recent memories will come from further down the bookcase, earlier in your life. Perhaps that's why sometimes you can so clearly visualise looking through the bars of your cot, and yet you can't remember what you had for breakfast.'

I pause and look up from my notes. All eyes are trained on me; my staff are holding their breath, waiting for me to finish.

'There is another part of the brain, another bookcase, separate from the first, more flimsy one. This bookcase is sturdy; it is your emotional bookcase. When dementia attempts to rock this one side to side, as if the two versions of you – before and after – are two tectonic plates that collide beneath the solid ground, this bookcase is stronger, more resilient, so the contents will be safer for longer. Even though you may forget that your friends or family visited recently – because that book comes off your factual bookcase – what stays with you are the feelings you had of love, happiness and comfort when they were near. You may forget what you did, what you spoke about or that they even popped by, but you know you feel safe and happy when you see them. So even if they don't appear to remember, don't ever stop visiting those with dementia ...'

I stop then, swallowing hard. I look up at the room; eight pairs of eyes stare back.

'The reason why I'm telling you all this is because I've just been diagnosed with Alzheimer's myself.' I pause then, giving it time to sink in. 'But I know you can help me.'

I see many visibly relax in their chairs as I say that, a call to arms. They know as much as I do that I'd never want to be seen as a victim. But there is silence as I stare back at them from the front. Some people have their heads down, and from others I see that sympathetic stare, their heads cocked gently to the side. They don't know how to react. I get that; I didn't either.

I smile my biggest smile. 'I can see I've shocked you all into silence,' I say. 'Well, that's a first.'

I ask the first group not to mention my diagnosis, and then the second group filter into the room and I repeat the same session, concluding with the bit where I tell them about my own diagnosis. Again the reactions are mixed, most filing out of the room in silence. One of the other team leaders lingers after they've gone, then gives me a hug.

'That was very moving, Wendy,' he says. 'Are you OK?'

I nod. But it doesn't feel like it's about me right now.

I go back to my desk and email all my staff, letting them know that I'm here to answer any questions they might have, and then I leave for home, knowing that they will digest the news better when I'm gone, when they can talk about it between them openly, letting it sink in. But I have confidence in them, much more than I had in management. I know they'll come good.

I am not disappointed. Over the next few days the inventiveness of my staff lifts my spirits. They come up with a plan for each of them to have a different-coloured Post-it note assigned to them, so if they write a note on my desk I'll know instantly who it's from. As further clarification, they post their names on each colour and stick them to the whiteboard above my desk. Another person recognised that it might be confusing to keep calling me at different times on the days I work at home, so between them they work out a timetable that they'll only bother me with questions at a certain time of the day. They look to me to advise on when that time would be. And there are little things: instead of walking into my office as they usually would, I begin to notice they stop asking for immediate answers when they come in to ask something of me. Instead they just leave the question with me. 'Whenever you've got a minute ...' they say, removing any pressure on my brain to come up with something quickly. We even laugh about my dementia, a joke always making it seem less of a disaster. A few days later I wander into someone's office to ask if she's completed a task I've been waiting for.

'Er, I don't think you've asked me to do that,' comes the sheepish response. The others start giggling.

'As if Wendy would forget to ask you that!' someone says, letting me off the hook.

'Nice try,' I laugh. We all laugh.

The light is there, it's not all dark. I still know my time here is limited, but they make it easier to stay for a while longer.

I see the postman coming towards my house. The spring in his step has been swapped for a shuffle as the week has gone on. I watch as he heaves a pile of post from the red bag on his trolley and looks towards my house. I'm at the front door before he's pressed the bell. He holds out the bundle, thick with heavy books.

'For you again,' he sighs.

The smile of a few days ago when he'd handed me the first heavy bundle is long gone, replaced no doubt with backache. Since I found the page on the Alzheimer's Society website offering to send out free leaflets and books about a whole range of subjects on dementia, more and more have been arriving for me each day. I'd gone through the whole checklist, ticking every box in my desire for information – any information – that might tell me more. I rip open each envelope when he's gone, flicking through the titles: *Keeping Safe At Home, Talking To Your Children About Your Illness, Planning Ahead*. I put them in a pile on my coffee table; right now it's enough to have them nearby. A comfort blanket for darker days.

In the last few days I've started a blog called *Which Me Am I Today?* It's somewhere I can put all this new information I'm discovering and, most importantly, it serves as my memory when I know that each night my brain is deleting files as I sleep – the day before becoming as much of a mystery as the day ahead.

I still feel abandoned by the doctors who diagnosed me, so instead I scan the internet, my desire to learn more and more, to equip myself with something other than fear, pushing me on to click on more pages, to absorb everything I possibly can. The only thing, of course, is holding on to all that new information. I glance at the books on the coffee table.

It's been the same with every headline about dementia since I was diagnosed. I'd read one after another, my heart lifting at the thought of the miracle cure that most newspapers suggested might be on the horizon. I started taking vitamin E because it was claimed it could slow the progress of the disease. I stockpiled my cupboards, popping a pill into the daily box with all the others. But when one day I started to run out, I scoured the internet for more evidence, switching from tabloid newspaper headlines to research papers, and discovered there was little to prove it had any real effect. I threw the last empty bottle into the bin and didn't replace it.

Most newspapers will tell their readers that a healthy lifestyle helps prevent Alzheimer's, and I think of my old running shoes at the back of the wardrobe and remind myself not to believe everything I read. Now each headline fills me with a niggling disappointment instead of the hope it once did. I still want a cure, desperately. There's nothing wrong in hoping, but expecting – that just feels like pre-planned disappointment. Is it not better to live for today, just keeping in mind tomorrow? But then I think of my daughters: what if they were ever diagnosed with it?

There has to be something more that I can do. My eyes fall on another leaflet I've collected on my travels, *What To Do When A Potential Brain Donor Dies*. I shift in my chair; that's not what I mean. I want to do something now; I don't want to just sit here and wait for this disease to make its march on my mind. I balance my laptop on my knee and type in the details for the Alzheimer's Society, and that's when I see the words: *Be Involved*. I send an email, telling whoever will be reading it that I want to be involved as much as possible, while I still have the opportunity, feeling, as I type, the continuing sense of urgency that has settled itself inside me.

A few days later I open an email explaining that the Alzheimer's Society is putting together a national Join Dementia Research database, and they want to know whether I'd like to help raise awareness in Yorkshire. I know from my own findings that dementia research lags far behind that into cancer or heart disease, and the way of discovering more is to appeal for volunteers for studies, not just those with the disease, but their families, caregivers, and even people who simply want to help. I think of Gemma and Sarah again, and the hope of finding a cure in their lifetime, so I write back, explaining I'm happy to do anything.

The following week I'm on a train to London to receive media training. The idea is that with some training I'll know what to expect when journalists interview me and how to answer them, either in print, or on TV or radio. The world whizzes by at the windows and I feel thankful for the miles that pass between me and home, for the opportunity to be out in the world doing something, making a contribution instead of sitting idle and allowing this disease to spread not only through my own brain, but those of others. I think of all the people who have so tragically lost limbs or have had heart attacks and the technology that has been developed through research to help them, but what is there for dementia? We need those same brilliant brains to develop tools to help us with our memory, speech and cognitive problems so we can lead better lives. So we can *live* with Alzheimer's. I vow to say yes to anything I'm asked to do to help this cause.

That's how I find myself back on another train to London a few weeks later, a printed map of how to get to my destination in St Katharine's Dock and walking instructions from the Tube in my rucksack. I arrive early, as always, and sit quietly on a bench beside the River Thames. People and traffic rush by, seagulls flap their wings to keep up with passing tugboats, but I find peace in the stillness of the moment, an opportunity to be quiet inside and simply watch the world around me. Most of us spend idle moments pulling a phone from our pockets to fill the time, the art of observation waning every day. How strange that Alzheimer's has reminded me of the calmness to be found in a little time out when, simultaneously, I feel in a rush to make the most of every moment before it deserts me. Yet turning the sound down on the world, even for just a few minutes, can calm the racing mind and thoughts of the road ahead.

Today I'm going to the Alzheimer's Society headquarters to hear more about joining the Research Network. Normally you have to be a member of the network for six months before you can join, but I had written to the network research manager a few weeks before telling him I couldn't wait that long to be of assistance. *If I wait six months, I might not be capable*, I'd told him. That feeling of urgency striking again, of wondering just what my shelf life would be, my 'use by' date indeterminable. I know my time at work is coming to an end, so maybe voluntary work like this will fill the space. Thankfully the Research Network people agreed to forego the six-month rule.

The Research Network matches 'monitors' with researchers who are carrying out new studies or drug trials into the disease. As a monitor, results are fed back to you so you can assess that the funding is being spent and allocated correctly. More importantly, it gives you the opportunity to hear about the trials from the researchers at regular intervals. It must be a lonely job being a researcher sometimes, so having the chance to listen to them is an exciting prospect. Being a monitor sounds perfect for me, a way for my diseased brain to still feel useful, and to be one of the first to hear about new areas of research.

At the head office, I'm shown into a room where for a second the noisy chatter distracts and unnerves me. I get a cup of tea and sit at the edge of the room so I can watch for a while, taking it all in, distinguishing voices and conversations. People soon come over to say hello, no one knowing I have dementia of course – to them I could be anyone, a researcher or carer – and I'm grateful for a moment that this disease doesn't show on the outside. When the meeting starts, everyone sits down, and we go around the table introducing ourselves.

'I'm living with dementia and I'm here today because I want to learn more about research,' I tell the room. I notice the eyes that hold my gaze for a moment longer, the pause before the next person speaks, the curiosity;

perhaps they, just like me, forget that Alzheimer's isn't something you can see.

Everyone takes their turn. One man who cares for his mum introduces himself, telling the room his mum '*really* has dementia'. He catches my eye and it feels as if somehow he's saying that my case isn't real.

'Well, dementia has to start somewhere,' I tell him. 'There is a beginning as well as a middle and an end, and I'm someone at the beginning.'

He looks back at me, surprised, as if he's never thought of that before, which seems strange to me until I remind myself that only 5 per cent of people diagnosed with dementia have young-onset Alzheimer's, so he wouldn't be expecting to see me sitting at the table alongside him. I remind myself of the first image that I'd held in my mind about someone with Alzheimer's and suddenly his reaction makes perfect sense.

Do you remember that last cigarette? When you finally realised it was now or never? It might surprise you to know that I do. How strange the choice the mind makes, the memories it holds fast. That it can still see so clearly that last blue smoke curling up from your face, and yet it can't tell me who came to visit yesterday. You must remember peeling back the cellophane, feeling the tiny resistance as you pushed up the lid, removed the foil paper, took the perfect white stick from the packet, the others collapsing into the space it left behind.

You'd started smoking back in college, bizarrely to try and convince someone else to stop. But your addictive personality had clung to you, hanging around year after year. You grew apart slowly, found you had less and less in common; for you it was that tiny individual, the guilt you felt smoking with a baby in the house, and then the tightening in your chest that meant it was harder and harder to get your breath back when running around after a toddler. The next baby was just a seed of a thought, yet surely you were strong enough to kick the habit before another tiny being entered your world. You'd tried before to say goodbye, stepping away slowly to ease the pain, but that last time, it was going to be different. A swifter departure than you'd tried before. You lit the last cigarette, dragged on it and saw the end burn bright orange; you inhaled deeply, and then released a great plume of smoke into the air. And that was it. The end. You stubbed it out and threw the last nineteen away with it.

The smell clung to you long after they hit the bottom of the bin, and that bitter taste at the back of your throat, you'd never noticed before, not until you'd fallen out of love with its seductive effects. Within days your food tasted nicer, within weeks the tightness in your chest had gone. You bought new trainers and a new gym kit, and exercise became your new addiction, feeling positive replaced your need for nicotine. Years later, running became your new obsession as you enjoyed the feeling of completing a 10 km race, the friendly faces that lined the street to cheer you on better company than the smoke that had once filled your lungs. But, curiously, you never forgot that last cigarette just like the addiction, the memory has clung on tight inside me too. It's hard to fathom now when there are so many 'lasts' you'd rather exchange for that. If only we could pick and choose the files that get deleted, if we could swap a last cigarette for something else: the last run, the last cake baked, the last drive in your beloved silver Suzuki. But you didn't know then they would be lasts, dementia gave you no warnings. Not like the last cigarette, the one that marked the change to a healthier lifestyle, a change that should see you fit and well long into your retirement. But that was a decision you made for yourself. No one else made it for you.

It is Sunday afternoon and I'm ironing at home in front of the TV. There's an Agatha Christie murder mystery just about to start, an old black-and-white one, I can't remember the title, but I know instinctively it's one that's a favourite. I pick up the first blouse in my pile, one eye on the iron, one on the telly, just the way it's always been. A new character enters the scene, or at least I think it's a new character. *Were they in the last scene?* By the time I've worked it out, they're gone. I put the iron down, squinting at the TV, my brow furrowed above my glasses. Who is this new character? Have I seen them before? This doesn't feel right.

I feel anxiety rise in my chest, swelling with the heat of the steam from the iron. I remember then many

Sundays, lost under a pile of ironing while I worked out 'whodunnit' on the box before anyone else, weekends when Sarah or Gemma might say, 'How did you know?' when I got there before them. But this, this is different. I can't keep up, there are too many characters, the plot is moving too fast, it's too confusing. I switch the television off with the remote control and stand staring at the black screen, a fuzzy outline of my own reflection staring back. This normally relaxing activity has suddenly lost its appeal. It's like this all the time now. I'm unable to follow plots of programmes and films, forgetting all the little clues that are laid down along the way. I'll be watching something when suddenly I can hear all these questions in my head: *Who are they? Where did they come from? Have they been in it before?* One question quickly followed by another, yet no one to ask. I realise then that the sighs of impatience are coming from me.

It's strange, but I've noticed that I can watch films that I've seen dozens of times before, the ones requiring little concentration, the ones with songs that break up and lighten the narrative, the ones where I know the characters as if they're old friends, the places as if I've walked those streets myself. Not that I can remember what happens – it's always a surprise at the end – but I feel a certain familiarity throughout, a sense of the ending, even if I don't remember the details. It isn't stressful to watch those films, and every time is a little like the first. Perhaps that's a benefit of dementia. I've noticed that there are some upsides, like the series on television that I long not to end; for me it's *The Great British Bake Off*. Who doesn't enjoy that sense of escapism it offers, where little matters apart from the correct measurements for a perfect batter or springy sponge, where the worst sin is a soggy bottom? For me now, it never ends. Instead, when I get to the series finale, the winner is always a surprise to me, and then I go right back to the first episode and settle down in front of the TV with a cup of Yorkshire tea and get to know the contestants all over again.

There was a time when a pile of novels always graced my bedside table, when the last thing I heard at night before I drifted off was the soft thud of 300 pages landing on my carpet. But the same book has been beside my bed for the last few months, the page folded at exactly the same place, the characters stuck in a storyline that hasn't moved on. I've found myself reading and re-reading the same few pages, the plot never quite sticking in my head until I've given up altogether. It was hard giving up reading. I used to love getting lost in a good book. And yet, I knew there must be an alternative, that I didn't have to let it go altogether. Does it have to be so black and white, or could there be a middle ground? And then it came to me: I would switch from novels to short stories. I've never read many before, but they are more manageable, the characters who live for just a few pages sticking more firmly in my head, the anxiety of trying to remember their back story gone from my chest. Reading is a pleasure again, now that I've thought of a way to adapt.

When I find an alternative action or way of thinking, of working around this disease that has taken over my brain, it feels less like the world is closing in around me and more instead that new opportunities are opening up, that there are ways of living with dementia, that far from a full stop, the beginning of the end, it can be just a comma. I can swap novels for short stories, delighting in the words on the page instead of the plot itself. I've found myself rediscovering the delights of poems, of books that I used to read the girls when they were tiny. There are the losses, but there are also the gains, and for another fleeting moment I realise that a progressive illness can focus the mind in a very special way. That thought has been coming to me a lot lately.

Another click on the research tab on the Join Dementia Research website, this time a clinical trial I've signed up for. I'd applied not thinking of adverse effects – after all, what could be worse than Alzheimer's itself? So now there are two very friendly women sitting in my living room and Sarah is making tea for us all in the kitchen.

They asked for her to be here – I wasn't too sure why at the time – but when she sits down, the steam from the cups weaving in and out of our conversation, I understand why. They are here to explain more about the trial. It is nicknamed MADE: Minocycline in Alzheimer's Disease.

'This trial aims to determine whether minocycline is superior to a placebo in affecting the disease course over a two-year period in patients with very early Alzheimer's disease,' one of the ladies explains to Sarah. She nods, but I notice the look that passes between us. 'Researchers will measure whether the drug is effective in reducing the rate of decline in cognitive and functional outcomes.'

Sarah shifts in her seat and looks at me as the woman continues to explain to her how minocycline is traditionally used as a treatment for acne, but studies have shown that its anti-inflammatory effects could be effective in Alzheimer's because it has the ability to cross the blood-brain barrier.

'Now, let's have a look at the paperwork,' the second lady says, shuffling some papers in her lap. I notice that all the forms she has to complete are on behalf of the 'carer', and now I realise why Sarah is here. I sit up a little taller in my chair, wanting to be noticed, understanding that they have perhaps been unsure whether I am capable of making the decision to be part of the trial myself. Another example of how health professionals overlook the person sitting in front of them, dismissing them as a 'sufferer', writing them off with their diagnosis. But I am determined to be heard. And so I ask questions, lots of them, this brain that still works so well on good days set on proving to them why I've chosen to take part in this trial, to understand more about this disease, to empower myself. The more I talk, the more control I take back. I tell them Sarah is here as my daughter, not my carer, as I live alone. They look suitably embarrassed and they apologise. Then they look at me when they answer. I instantly like these ladies much more. They explain that on the two-year trial there are three options: the 400 mg dose, the 200 mg dose or the placebo.

'I don't want the placebo,' I joke, knowing I don't have a choice in the matter. This isn't why I want to take part: I hope the trial shows the drugs work. I sign the forms, we come to an agreement that they'll never refer to Sarah as my carer again, and then they leave.

It is three weeks later and the drugs arrive along with Lisa, the research administrator. She unpacks the first three months of the trial tablets on my kitchen table. For some reason they are in giant packets and my hands look tiny as I pick them up and turn them over to read each side of the packet. Over the next few weeks I take them each day, obsessed at first with working out if my head feels any clearer, if my memory is sharper. It will be two years before I find out if I've been taking a placebo, but along with the tablet something else has been planted inside my belly, a little seed that will start to grow, a curiosity about research and learning more and more about this disease. That in itself starts to sprout a new feeling, a sense of purpose, of hope, of once again being valued, of taking back some of what dementia has stripped away from me.

The bus is speeding along. Streets and cars and people whizzing by at the windows. And I can't hear anything except the thudding of my heart in my chest. I try again.

'Could you just stop here?' I say.

'No. The next stop is two miles away.'

There it is again. The anxiety rising from deep inside.

I've been using buses more and more since I got my bus pass, a benefit of Alzheimer's, but sometimes I get easily confused by the numbers on the front. I think one is the number I want, then find myself travelling through streets going the opposite way from my destination. I get off, shake my head, wonder how I'd got so mixed up. Other buses don't always stop at the same stop. So, like today, I'd pressed the bell when I'd realised that I'd got on the wrong bus.

'But I need to get off,' I say to the driver. There's little I can do to disguise the panic in my voice, and already my mind is trying to catch up, trying to think fast enough. Where is the bus heading? How far is two miles? Where will I need to get off? How will I get back? I'm standing in the aisle on the bus, my pleas for the driver to stop falling on deaf ears. I feel every bump in the road. I'm jostled around as my feet try to stay firm. And then I see a young man trying to catch my eye, a friendly smile. He stands up and walks towards me.

'Are you OK?' he asks.

'I'm not sure,' I say. 'I missed my stop. I don't know how to get back. I've got Alzheimer's. I sometimes get the numbers on the bus mixed up.'

'Don't worry,' he says. 'I'll show you where to get the bus back again.'

He's reassuring, calm. I trust him. I sit down and the tightness inside eases a little. But my mind is still spinning and I'm still trying to work it out myself: where I am, how to get back. When at last the bus pulls into a stop, the driver calls from his cabin: 'You should take more notice next time!'

I feel silly, confused – and sad too. I know that York is aiming to be a dementia-friendly city. Most bus drivers are wonderful; perhaps he was off work the day they handed out the dementia training. The young man shows me to the stop where I can get a bus back home. I thank him.

'Hopefully next time I'll get the right bus,' I say.

'Hopefully next time you'll get the right driver,' he replies, waving me off.

***

I'm nervous walking into the lecture theatre – the room seems huge, the ceiling high. There are no windows, and just low lighting. There are dozens of voices bouncing off the walls, a sea of new faces. A fuzzy memory that the old me would have strolled in confidently. I feel Sarah at my side; her nursing studies lecturer is also here to support both of us today. This is my first dementia conference, part of York's Women of the World (WOW) Festival, and also the first time meeting face to face with other women with dementia. I scan the room. There must be eighty people in here and only six of them have dementia. I try to work out which ones they are, studying their faces, their clothes, before realising how ridiculous that idea is. Do *I* look like I have dementia? Do any of us? It's not a disease we have stamped on our foreheads; it is an invisible disability.

One of the organisers steps forward and introduces herself. I instantly feel more relaxed as she leads us to our seats at the front. I ask Sarah if I can sit on the end of the row so I don't feel trapped. There's something else, though, aside from the unfamiliarity, that's causing the tight ball deep inside my stomach – it's the thought of sharing, of speaking out. I look at all the faces of strangers around me, the sheer size of the room, and wonder if I'm ready to open up to them about life with dementia, how much I'll be expected to share. I've never been a talker, only a listener. The handful of best friends

I've had over my lifetime could always sit and chat to me for hours about their problems, knowing I'd listen, that I'd never repeat a word, but they rarely heard mine in return. The thought of sharing with all these people is daunting.

The lights go down and a range of experts take to the front of the stage. Most of what is discussed first goes over my head, so instead I focus on my surroundings and relax into my chair. It's enough that I'm here – I don't need to worry about keeping up. But then the next speaker is announced and my mind snaps back into focus. It's Agnes Houston, who was diagnosed with young-onset dementia in 2006. I sit up straight as she speaks so eloquently about her experience. She was diagnosed ten years ago and is still so composed, so articulate that my heart swells with hope inside. By the time she leaves the stage, I'm clapping louder and more furiously than anyone else in the room; she has inspired me. Now I pay closer attention. The next person up is talking about getting rid of self-service tills in the supermarkets. I'm desperate to call out, to say I like them, that they give me time to go at my own pace, so I don't feel rushed. But what is the etiquette here? I hesitate and then the moment is gone, the private me letting me down, too nervous to make my voice heard. I sigh, deflated, knowing Agnes would never allow herself to go unheard.

An hour or so later, the six of us with dementia are invited into a room for a round-table discussion. It's a much nicer room with windows and a view out over the university gardens and their perfectly green lawns. We introduce ourselves. There are women from all walks of life: doctors, academics, women just like me. All of their stories are so different, but my diagnosis is the newest. Some of them were diagnosed ten or even fifteen years ago, but here they are, sitting around the same table with me, chatting eloquently about their lives and what they find difficult. We laugh too, especially when we describe the same challenges, not needing to explain how it *really* feels, just knowing from a short description. We agree that if a thought pops into our heads we're allowed to share it straight away rather than risk it vanishing – we all know what that feels like – and again there are peals of laughter. The more we speak, the more hope grows inside me, the thought that in ten or fifteen years there's every chance I could still be like them. I am determined to share more, to see the nods that come back to me, to know that someone else feels the same.

At one point we start talking about the government's role in supporting provision, and another woman speaks up, talking about how Margaret Thatcher could do more to help. A couple of us glance at one another – David Cameron is prime minister, and has been for five years – but nobody corrects her. What difference does it make? We know what she means. Instead we continue the conversation, feeling at ease, more like we're with family than other women we've only just met. There are the stories of loss and abandonment, of those who haven't understood us, but mostly we laugh. Dementia isn't winning in that room – we are. When we file out for lunch, I feel more empowered than I have done in months.

You were never academic; sport was always your thing. At school you were captain of all the sports teams – tennis, hockey, netball – it felt like the only thing you were good at, so you were determined to be the best. You liked the challenge. Some things never change.

You weren't clever enough for university – or so you were told – instead you were advised to go to PE college. At first you loved it simply because you loved sports so much, but being away from home, you needed to swap family for friends, and something didn't click. You didn't enjoy the parties, you found it hard to mix, and it marked you out as different. Only a little, but that's sometimes all it takes. There are always girls who will say horrible things about you, who will isolate you if you give them half the chance and, having never experienced this before, you couldn't cope. You dropped out of college and people became your enemy for a long time. If you stayed alone, you wouldn't get hurt; that's what logic told you at the time. But then you were only young, still in your teens. Is it any wonder that you

stopped opening up? That you became a private person, one who
would never share, never talk about her feelings. Someone so
different from me?

A different room, a different discussion. It's the afternoon
of the WOW conference and this time there are only two
of us with dementia around the table; the rest are healthcare professionals: university lecturers, researchers, care
specialists. But I feel less confident now. Sarah sits beside
me. She's been part of the nursing 'bank', working shifts
in different care homes, and making notes about the best
and worst things about them. We've joked that she's
checking them all out for a time when I will need them,
but sitting here around this table, that discussion feels
very real. She shares with the group some of the things
she's observed. I'm proud to hear her speak out. I can
see how much she cares and I know that's partly because
of me. But inside my stomach is a tight knot, increasing
whenever anybody mentions poor care, lack of choices,
even abuse in care homes. *Is this really my future?* I feel
frightened, feeble and impotent. I sit listening, overwhelmed by dark feelings. How different it feels now
from the discussion this morning with the other women
who have dementia: how strong and empowered we
felt, despite the disease. Here, though, we are silent, an
idea perpetuated around the table of us shuffling along
towards the end of our lives, hopeless and helpless, on

some kind of conveyor belt just ticking off the stops that society dictates we should have before we topple off the end altogether. And then the other lady with dementia speaks out.

'Well, I've already booked my place at Dignitas,' she says. 'When I can't take care of myself any more, I'm not going to put myself into the hands of a care home that can't look after me properly, so when the time comes I'll go to the euthanasia clinic in Switzerland and end my own life.'

The rest of the room falls silent. I find myself nodding in agreement, but then glance at Sarah from the corner of my eye; her head is down. Guilt stings inside at the thought she caught me nodding, but I can't deny that this has been the most empowering statement I've heard all day. With any progressive illness it's the lack of control that's the hardest thing to live with. For me, if I can find a way of living with dementia, shouldn't I be allowed to find a way of dying with it too? It's not a conversation I thought I'd be having in my head today. This morning the conversation between us six women focused on what we *could* do, but this afternoon it feels like decisions are taken out of our hands – unless we claim them back like the woman who insists she's going to Dignitas. I admire her for already making that decision, particularly as I shuffle out of the room feeling so despondent, frustrated, detached and in despair about my own future.

But in the days that have followed, the conversation about euthanasia has repeatedly returned to me. I'd never had to consider it seriously before and yet I'd immediately agreed with what that lady had said. I'd watched both of my parents die from cancer, and it was only natural, as I'd seen them suffer, that I'd wished I could end their pain. But with regards to me, that was something I'd never considered. I admired that woman's conviction, her determination to end her life in Switzerland, her way. But I could never do that. I could never ask my girls to travel with me because just the thought of them travelling back alone is enough to break my heart. And so it's the illegality of euthanasia that I find so frustrating, the fact that another decision has been taken out of my hands – this time by the laws of the land. It's when I think like this, when I don't feel like I have control, or rights, that I start feeling panicky inside. When all the *what ifs* or *what about whens* come rushing up from my gut and squeeze the words right out of my mouth; when the tears prick the back of my eyes; when I feel scared. What will happen to me when I go over the edge into that person I don't know? Will I be blissfully unaware? Will I not even recognise the pain written across the two faces that mean the most to me – Sarah and Gemma? Euthanasia would save us all from that.

The wind is brushing my hair, the ground moving beneath me. I look to my right at the river rushing by alongside me, and the faces speeding past in the opposite direction on the path. We say hello, I wobble slightly, but this feels like freedom, like independence, more like me. It's a similar feeling to running again, except it's not my feet that are hitting the pavement, but the wheels of my new pink bike. Getting outside, into the fresh air, connects me to a place where dementia doesn't exist, just space and a big sky above me.

I'd been out for a sunny walk with Sarah when we'd seen signs for a bicycle festival in Rowntree Park. We followed the river path into the park and there was a circle of colourful tents all displaying bikes for sale. We ambled round with no intention to buy and then I'd seen it, this bright pink bike propped up, an old-fashioned wicker basket strapped to the front, a brown leather seat and handlebar grips. It was perfect.

'Are you sure?' Sarah had said, but before she'd had a chance to question me, I'd paid the man and even picked out a pink bell and helmet to match. I wasn't particularly a fan of pink, but I knew I'd never lose it, or forget which one was mine with such bright paintwork.

Today is my first proper run out on it. I'd been a bit wobbly to start with, but a few minutes down the road I'd found the rhythm of the bike and got to grips with the brakes. As the world rushes past, I remember how painful it had been to give up my driving licence, but somehow this takes some of the hurt away and as I cover more ground my confidence grows. I remember how driving had become impossible, the speed of the car not giving me enough time to process, to work out what to do before a junction, but this bike moves more slowly, buys me more time for my brain to catch up. I see the junction approaching and I pull on the brakes. Everything is going well. I go to turn right, and then something happens, a disconnect. The next thing I know I'm on the tarmac, gravel biting into my flesh, stinging pain, a moment's disorientation. I'm in a crumpled heap, bruised and confused. *How did that happen?* I pick myself and the bike up off the road, and look around. Thankfully it's quiet; there are no cars. I know I've been lucky. I limp home, wheeling my bike at my side, going over and over what happened. There must have been a pothole in the road, something that caught the wheel and made me lose balance.

A few days later I know I need to get back in the saddle. I try again, this time more tentatively, but then I feel the breeze beneath my helmet, the world whizz by, and my confidence returns. There *must* have been something in the road before. The same junction approaches. I scan the tarmac, but I see nothing. I go to turn right and the same thing happens, a disconnect somewhere, faulty wiring. I pull myself up off the road. Again, I'm lucky. What is it about my brain that means I can't turn right? It's not just the car, but the bike too. I look at my new pink bike, the perfect paintwork now scratched from my two falls, and my heart sinks. There must be a way of outwitting this disease, of keeping this freedom.

My bike stands motionless for days while I think about it, and then it comes to me: a route to the shops and home where I only need to take left-hand turns. I can do this in one big circle. I pull on my helmet and take the handlebars of my bike, wheeling it out into the road and climbing on. As I swing my leg over the saddle, there is that moment's hesitation, an anxiety that tries to take hold inside, but I ignore it, knowing if I pay attention to every single knot in my stomach I'll be tied up for the rest of my life. I push away from the pavement and I'm off, that same light feeling in my ears, the world easing past, the smiles, the hellos from fellow cyclists, the nods of admiration for the outrageous colour of my bike. The first turn left approaches – easy. The second, the third, all of them done. I arrive at the shops and turn left to complete my circle and make it all the way home. As I approach home, my heart is racing, blood pounding at my temples, not with anxiety but with triumph. I climb off and prop my bike up against the wall.

There will be more rides out; there will be the rose tree and two bags of compost I balance in my basket, wobbling all the way home, hoping that Gemma and Sarah don't spot me and tell me off. There will be more of the outdoors, more freedom, independence. There will be all the journeys I take with a smile on my face, knowing I have outwitted Alzheimer's again.

I turn in the street, the crumpled map in my hand. I look from one end to the other. It all looks the same. But there is no sign, not the one I'm looking for, anyway. My breath swells hard inside my lungs and my throat constricts in response. *Deep breaths*, I tell myself. I walk more slowly this time, all the way up, all the way down. The café I'm looking for is still not here. I check the leaflet again. I had felt excited this morning when I left home to come to this dementia support group, excited and a little apprehensive, especially at the thought of walking in alone. I'd done up my dark blue parka before I left home, zipping over the hard anxious knot inside my tummy, and pulling the fur hood up to escape the cold. I'd arrived here, gearing up to walk in without anyone at my side, and then I'm lost. I check the leaflet again, and the map, then the street sign, the numbers; they seem to end at twenty-five. That can't be right. I walk back again, past tall buildings converted into flats and huge Georgian residences behind black iron railings, but there are no cafés here. I walk back up to the top and then it occurs to me that there is a junction with another road beyond. I cross over and yes, it is the same street, and when I look up there is the sign. Relief expands inside my lungs but now my hands are clammy and I feel stupid for not being able to find the place, so by the time I walk in, I'm flustered and nervous, but a smiling face greets me.

'I'm Emily,' she says, reaching out a hand and introducing me to the others. It takes me a few moments to put away the map, to explain that I got lost and confused, and then I look at all the faces staring up at me without judgement or criticism and remember that I'm in safe hands, that they understand – even if it was just a strange road design that got me all muddled up rather than the dementia.

I sit down and a chap called Damian makes me a cup of tea. He used to work for the Alzheimer's Society, Emily was a mental health nurse, and they set this group up because they saw there was a need for more dementia support in York. Each sip of hot tea that slips down my throat relaxes me more. I take my coat off and look around the table. There are only a handful of us and I'm definitely the youngest. The others are somewhere between sixty and eighty, and one lady in particular looks very quiet. She stares down into her lap, listening, but keeping herself to herself. I decide that I'll just listen today too, yet when people start to talk, I feel that same warmth that I did at the WOW Festival, a feeling of being amongst family, with those who know how it *really* feels to live with this new brain I'm still getting used to. But there's something else; Damian and Emily don't just want us to sit around and talk about what it's like to have dementia, they want us to help make the town a more friendly place for those with the disease.

'The council want to put together a new map of York for tourists,' Damian explains, handing out copies of the new proposed sign. 'They want us to ask you if you have any suggestions of how we can make it easier for someone with dementia to find their way around.'

My hunched, unsure body unfolds itself in the seat. I pick up the document and take a closer look.

'It needs some photographs,' someone says. 'To make it easier for people to identify where they are.'

I nod.

'And a clear "You Are Here" sign,' someone else says.

I nod again. 'Yes, definitely,' I say. So much for just listening. But it feels good to be asked.

We spend the next two hours like that, with Damian or Emily asking our opinions on lots of other things. If one of us gets something wrong or gets confused, there is no judgement. We can relax, speak and be heard. We feel validated, all of us around that table. By the time it is time to leave, it feels like a month is too long to wait until the next session. I smile and say goodbye to all the new friends I've made, and the lady who hasn't spoken throughout the entire meeting smiles back.

I walk home through York's cobbled streets, past tiny coffee shops serving scones and jam to tourists, feeling happy that we'd been able to offer something to help. There is something else, too, as I follow the path, the satisfaction that fear hasn't won the day, that I hadn't given up just because I couldn't find the café at first, or just because I was afraid to walk in alone. I know I have to keep pushing myself forward, to keep volunteering, to say yes to everything, to meet new people. Who knows what awaits me if I am brave enough.

I lost yesterday. I don't know what happened to it. People often ask me what it's like to have dementia on a bad day, but it's hard to remember; it's like I'm not there. Perhaps I don't want to acknowledge the days when Alzheimer's wins, when I go to bed and pull the duvet up over my ears because nothing about the world outside of me makes sense. It's like floating in and out of consciousness: one moment the world is in focus and I know exactly what I'm doing, the next it means nothing at all and I can't even say what I've just done. On those days I can *feel* the disease in my head, like it's eating away at all that is good in there, claiming more brain cells for its monstrous mission, stealing memory upon memory. On those days my head feels fuzzy and inflamed, as if it doesn't belong to me – and it doesn't, it's given over to the disease. I heard an analogy in a Dementia Friends session once, that the disease is like taking your Christmas tree lights out of the box each year; you unwind and untangle them, plugging them in to check for loose connections, and along the wire some tiny bulbs flash on and off, some don't come on at all, but you can't predict which ones are missing, the fault on the line, when or where it will occur.

On bad days, there is a fuzziness, similar to the way the picture on the telly looks when it starts to break up, making it harder to decipher. A fog descends, confusion reigns and there is no clarity from the moment I open my eyes. *Where am I?* My own handwriting on the note-pad beside my bed is a mystery, the words written by a stranger who slipped away while I slept. On those days there is little in my brain to help me through; it's as if it's been emptied overnight in my dreams, rebooted and restored to factory settings. Every day the alarms set on my iPad and in my phone remind me to take my medication. A simple task, something I do every single day, twice a day, and yet on bad days the alarm rings and it's as if I'm seeing it for the first time. Every single time. If there's no alarm, the task doesn't exist. On those days, there's a feeling I can liken to a fine necklace being all tangled up. I sit there for hours, trying to untangle the knots. To make my brain work hard to tell me the simplest of things. *What day is it? Have I set any reminders on my phone? Laid out any clothes that will give me clues?* If I'm feeling calm, I can sit there patiently and untangle the necklace, working out the reality of the day, or simply waiting for the fog to lift. But if panic rises in my throat, if it gets a hold of my heart, making it beat stronger and faster and louder, if I give in to it, then I become impatient with this metaphorical necklace and it takes all my strength not to throw it all over the floor, scattering thoughts like beads.

The key is always calm thoughts, waiting, looking at anything that distracts me from the fog; photographs in my memory room, a smiley face, a hill, a lake, a daughter.

It's not just what I can't see or fathom, it's what I *can* see, too. What I think is real, but is just an illusion designed to trick me by a brain gone AWOL on days like that. One morning I came downstairs and looked out at my back garden. My shed had gone; there was a blank where it once was, just a concrete base. Instead, a carpet tile lay on the fence. Perhaps it was the way the assailants hauled it out of my garden, my logical brain tried to reason. But then something cut through, more logically: a shed can't disappear. Can it?

I could have panicked then. I could have called the police and registered the crime. But instead I looked harder, wondering whether my mind was playing tricks on me. Instead I told myself I'd go back in thirty minutes; if it still wasn't there, I would know it was real. Later, the shed was there, of course it was. But this kind of thing happens a lot. There are sounds too. I have sat in my living room, relaxing in my chair, and the sound of gunshot has gone straight through me. I sit up in an instant, an ice-cold tingle shooting down my spine, my heart racing hard. But when I've looked outside and searched the streets for people fleeing, a road scattered with bodies, there has been nothing there, just folk going about their business. The gunshot nothing but a temporary short-circuit in my head. Just like the knocks on the door when no one is there.

I've learned to sit quietly on those bad days. I'll sit and watch the birds come and help themselves to breakfast in my garden. Their reliability brings normality to these confusing times. I can't always rely on what I can see or hear. Whatever I've seen is not always there; whatever I've heard doesn't always sound like that. Don't panic, just wait; it'll be OK. Logic has to win the day.

The one thing I remember about bad days is that I tell myself tomorrow will be better. It's not me: it's this cruel disease invading my head. At least I can still decipher the good days from the bad. I do wake up and wonder, *Which me am I today?* But at least I can still tell the difference, that's something to be thankful for.

I'm back on Tanner Row to return to the support group, and this time I find the café easily; the me who was last here helpfully circled the place on the map in biro. There is no fear or hesitancy as I walk in this morning, I might not remember the faces around the table, but I remember that I felt very relaxed around them. This time, as we sit around the table, we decide we want to come up with a catchy name for our group in the hope it will attract others. Many of us around the table make suggestions – all the usual culprits, those of us who are always first to speak up and now I include myself in that. I've found that saying 'yes' suits this new me, that being part of something, of decisions, of offering opinions, feels good inside. We've had one other meeting in between this and the first one, and I spoke up more then, but the lady I'd noticed before, the one who sits quietly, watching her hands in her lap, didn't say a word. She's here again today, though; perhaps she just likes the sense of being included. I can understand that.

We offer suggestions from each side of the table, brainstorming and going backwards and forwards, and then a tiny voice speaks. We all look up.

'How about Minds and Voices?' the usually silent lady says.

'I like that,' I say, and pride fills her face. I recognise in her a sense of achievement, of her heart filling with that feeling of being relevant in the room again; she grows in her chair in front of me.

Unanimously deciding to name the group York Minds and Voices, we come up with the strapline then: 'opening minds and moving forward'. That sums us up perfectly.

Between me and the stranger sitting at my dining table lies a small black video camera. Jim – a reporter for the BBC – has gone over how to use it several times, despite the fact I've got Sarah there as my memory. I've written down everything that he's said, and I know I've probably asked him the same question many times, but he's very patient, very good-humoured. He makes me feel calm and the black thing between us isn't half as scary as it was when he plonked it down, all wires and buttons. As I write down again where the power switch is – determined to remember everything myself – Sarah is asking him complicated questions about zooms and editing and all the Spielberg stuff.

When there's a pause between them, I stick my head up. 'Um, can you show me again how to switch it on and off?' I say.

It is January 2015 and Jim is here because the Hollywood film *Still Alice*, starring Julianne Moore as a woman diagnosed with young-onset Alzheimer's, is about to be released in the cinemas. The BBC's Victoria Derbyshire programme wants to make a short film to coincide with its release and they have given three of us living with dementia video cameras to record snippets of our everyday lives over a month.

There are many days when emails land from the Alzheimer's Society asking me if I would be interested in taking part in some interview or another. I say yes to everything while I can. I don't know how long I will have to take advantage of these new experiences, so I grab every one, even the ones I'm frightened of – *especially* the ones I'm frightened of. That's how I was put in touch with Jim. My job in this short film is to represent the early part of the disease, Keith Oliver will show the middle stage, and a man called Christopher Devas will represent the late stage, with his wife Veronica filming for him.

When Jim leaves, the equipment he's left behind sits staring at me from the table. Occasionally I take a closer look, a hand tentatively wandering across the buttons. I jump back when it springs to life. It's now or never, I tell myself, taking a deep breath. I pick up the camera and start walking around my house, talking into the microphone, recording the front of the fridge with my calendar pinned to it showing what I'm doing that week. Or at least I thought I was filming. When I finish, I go to 'play back' and realise I had forgotten to press 'record'. I try again, and this time the mic is the wrong way round, but the video camera feels more comfortable in my hand, and despite getting it wrong, my confidence is growing.

The third time, I record everything I want to; my pillbox labelled with days of the week, a selection of brightly coloured tablets filling each little compartment like sweeties. My memory room and all the photos that make me feel calm, the box of memories I keep in there, complete with Sarah and Gemma's tiny first shoes on top. I talk on camera about my greatest fear – the day that I don't recognise my daughters.

'I've said to them that one day you'll come in the room and I won't know who you are,' I confide to the camera. 'I won't know your name, but I'm sure I'll feel that emotional connection of love that we have for each other. And for them to always recognise that even though I won't recognise them, I still love them.'

I put the camera down. Some bits that I'm sharing, the fears deep down inside, are harder than I realised. I take a moment, a few slow breaths, and then remind myself that this film will help people to understand more about dementia. I switch it on again. I'm as honest as I can be, knowing that Jim will take the snippets he needs when the four weeks are up.

The next day I sit on the bus to work, the camera in my rucksack. I've got up extra early because I want to film before anyone else arrives. The office is in darkness when I get there, the last of the night still clinging to the windows. I want to record that moment when I got lost in my office, when I walked out of the door and didn't have a clue where I was. I press 'record' and see the red light start flashing, but when I begin to speak, the words are lost. I go back to my desk and write a little script, something I can read as I'm walking. I start again, leaving the safety of my office, just like I had on that day, and stepping out into the corridor and, as I hear my voice, echoing down the emptiness of the hallways, I feel my heart start to thud under my blouse. As if it's happening again. The tiny image in the viewfinder brings back that day that had twisted my insides with a fear like no other I'd ever experienced. I feel again the sense of loss within myself, a complete detachment from my own mind. It's terrifying.

I pause in the corridor. Despite the fact I'm reading from a script, my thumping heart threatens to steal the words written in biro. I take one tentative step and then another, an almost exact carbon copy of that day. I go through two sets of doors, then into the bathroom with its safety glass, into the soft pink of the toilet cubicle, and there for a few moments I stay, just as I had on that day. I stop recording and take a breath or two, blood thumping at my temples, the camcorder in standby mode, the soft whirr of the mechanisms still turning over. I leave the cubicle, grateful for the cool air that hits me back in the corridor, of the recognition that greets me. This day is *not* like the last.

I hurry back to my desk and push the camcorder back into my bag, but I know for sure then the impact this film will have, and the anxiety is replaced with a feeling of empowerment. I have always been so private, so protective of sharing anything personal, and yet I know that by sharing I can change opinions, I can shift the images instilled in people's minds of what it's like to have dementia, like the elderly person in a bed, the same pictures that flooded my own brain when the word had been first mentioned. I can show that dementia has a beginning and a middle, as well as an end.

A few weeks later the Alzheimer's Society sends me another email, this time asking if I will review *Still Alice* for them before its cinema release. Of course I say yes. It arrives special delivery and the postman hands over a white Jiffy bag and inside the DVD of *Still Alice*, the fictional tale of a fifty-year-old linguistics professor diagnosed with dementia. I hold the package tightly between my fingers; I know it's not going to be an easy watch. I had already read the book three times, the advantage of having Alzheimer's myself meaning that the plot unveiled itself surprisingly every single read, but while I'd been impressed with how accurate it was – each of my worst fears unfurling at the turn of the page – I'd been able to put down the book when it became too much. But watching it on film, seeing an animated version of the character I'd felt so much for in the book and a straight run-through of her decline, is going to be hard.

It feels safer somehow to watch it while the sun still shines through my window in the early afternoon. I slip the DVD into the player and wait for the credits to roll. In my lap I have a notepad and pen, *I'll write notes,* I tell myself as the first scenes unfold. *I'll detach*, I promise. *Be professional, not personal.* One of the first scenes is of Alice jogging around her university campus. I smile, remembering my own runs. I think of the trainers at the back of the wardrobe and a sadness swells inside, but before I know it, Alice has stopped, the world spins around her, out of control, the buildings she clearly knows so well suddenly unrecognisable. I see the blank on her face, the disorientation, and the likeness immediately takes me back to that office corridor. I can feel the pen relax inside my clammy palm, but I can't tear my eyes away from the film.

A few scenes on, Alice is delivering a speech; she stumbles over a word, shrugging off the problem in the same way I had. I'm staring at the screen, watching scenes unfold in front of me as if they are plucked from my own life. I don't move; it feels as if the very breath has been stolen from me, as if breathing is nothing more than an inconvenience, a distraction from what has captivated me so much. I don't realise I've been holding my breath until I hear a long, deep sigh. It's the end of the school day and I can hear chatter outside my windows, the beep of the pedestrian crossing as parents ferry their children home, but my eyes stay fixed on the screen.

The image of a butterfly folder grabs my attention. In it, Alice has put instructions on how to take her own life when she goes over the edge into someone she doesn't know. But her pitiful dilemma unfolds on screen: how do you know when you're standing on the edge waiting to fall? We all like to think we'll know, that we can rely on the conscious mind we use to make decisions to remind us, but one of my greatest fears is played out on screen like a moment from the future fast forwarded to meet me right here as Alice desperately tries to carry out the instructions her healthier self has left her, but the cruelty of time has already taken her beyond that point of no return.

During another scene a few moments on, when the disease has made its march and her younger daughter has become an unfamiliar face, my breath comes in short wisps and my head feels too light for my shoulders. I've read about this moment. I've attempted to conjure up images too painful to linger on, but here is the hurt being played out in front of me. My eyes are fixed on Alice, the way she looks at her daughter, the glazed stare in her eyes; Julianne Moore has got it just right. It's only then that I step out of the film, reminding myself that Moore is playing this woman, but how has she got it so right? Her character is looking directly at her daughter and yet it's clear she doesn't *see* her.

By the time the film ends, as the credits roll and the player dispatches the DVD from the machine, the notebook is still lying open in my lap, the pen in my hand, not a single word written down.

I need a cup of tea. I get up from my chair, my body stiff, my mind rolling a series of images, all sensation given way to a nothing numbness. I stare out of the window, watch the birds hopping around my garden on tiny slender legs until my brain returns to me. I know I need to watch it again, so I push the DVD back into the machine, and sit down with notepad and pen.

As I rewatch the opening scenes, an intelligent, afflu-ent woman celebrating her birthday with her family, I write: *It captures the reality that Alzheimer's shows no bias of age, sex, intelligence, wealth or ethnicity when selecting those to challenge with the disease.* But a few scenes on, Alice's eyes hold my attention again – is this what Gemma and Sarah see when they look at me on a bad day? And my mind flashes forward, images crash into my brain of days when I constantly wander around with that blankness writ-ten large on my face, when those are the eyes my girls know, when they've forgotten about these eyes that see them back. Suddenly, I feel panicked. I don't want my daughters to ever be my carers; I want to be their mum ... *I want to be their mum*. The scenes whizz by in the film and I snap myself back into concentrating. Under the last sentence I write four words: *powerful, shocking, raw, inevitability*. Then before I know it, the player has ejected the DVD again. I look up at the windows at the end of my second attempt. Traffic rumbles by and it's still light, for now.

I make another cup of tea and try again. What is so fascinating for me about this film is the way it captures the true picture of the disease from the pre-diagnosis stage and the slow, barely noticeable decline. I remember the questions without answers that accompany those endless days – searching and fearing the explanations in equal measure. The film shows how memory is stripped away so indiscriminately, and that no amount of love we feel for someone can protect against the theft of our recognition of them. But the emotion must remain, even when there's a space where their name should be. Surely that much love can't just disappear? It must stay trapped inside instead. I make a note on my pad to tell the girls this, to make sure they know. Has that thought occurred to me before?

Everyone remembers that feeling of losing a precious possession, an item of sentimental value. If you're old enough, it's happened many times throughout your life, and if you're a toddler it's the most traumatic thing that's ever occurred. For those of us with Alzheimer's this is our everyday, yet it's not items that disappear, but our most precious memories, the stories that make up who we are. But we don't lose our emotions, so the love must just be locked away behind those sad, glazed eyes.

I watch the film over again one more time. I write in my notes how impressed I am by how refreshingly real Alice's decline is, how her story is portrayed with sensitivity, avoiding clichés. It is a powerful insight into dementia, the reality of the disease, the reality of the effects it has on the individual and those around them. It is a shockingly accurate reflection of my own experience. And that hurts and heartens me equally.

By the time the player ejects the DVD for a third time, the night is black, the screen goes blank. I sit alone in the dark.

Another email, another request, another 'yes' mailed back to the Alzheimer's Society, but this time much more enthusiastically than any before, because it was an invitation inviting me to attend the premiere of *Still Alice* in London. I've travelled down on my own, getting here early so that I know where I need to be in good time, outwitting the panic that always threatens to descend with dementia. I find the Curzon cinema, but the doors are locked and bolted and beyond them is darkness. It is hours yet until the stars will start to arrive, but at least I know where I need to be. Instead I wander the streets of Mayfair in the smart camel coat I've bought especially, my Dementia Friends forget-me-not badge pinned proudly to the lapel.

I find a café nearby and sit down for a cup of tea, watching people come and go; the businessmen flitting in and out between meetings, the tourists clutching maps of the city, friends shopping for the day, making space between the tables and chairs for their huge bags with designer names stamped on the front. Sometimes it still feels incredible to find myself here, alone in a café in London, far from my office up in Yorkshire, the intensely private person in me buried under the avalanche of a disease that is so perversely opening up new opportunities to me every single day, new experiences that I grab with both hands because it has also granted me the gift of having a better sense of how short life is. I sip my tea and smile, at odds with my diseased brain and yet strangely thankful for it. Can something so terrible as the diagnosis of a progressive illness really be seen as a good thing?

I turn my attention instead to my itinerary for the day. First I'll be meeting Christopher and his wife Veronica, who also took part in the filming for the Victoria Derbyshire programme. I'm going to be meeting Angie, a dementia support worker, and Gillian, who she supports. I know from my experiences at the WOW Festival and

York Minds and Voices that meeting others with dementia always makes me feel safe, so I'm confident they'll
help keep the nerves at bay before we meet Julianne
herself. I hadn't even heard of her before I was told about
this film, but Sarah had been so excited, telling me she's
a big Hollywood star and one of her favourite actresses,
and so inside my rucksack are two copies of the novel,
which I've promised to get signed for my daughters.

Finally, the hands roll around the café's clock face and
it's time to head back to the cinema. Another new experience, another lonely walk into a room. It's impossible
to ignore the butterflies bunched inside my coat. When
I arrive at the cinema, the area has been transformed;
it's not quiet like it was a few hours ago. Instead, railings
prevent anyone from getting into the cinema, paparazzi
and their ladders are a few feet deep, spilling into the road,
and beyond them there's a flash of red at their feet – the
carpet for the stars. I stand watching for a few moments
as the panic I'd been so desperate to avoid this morning
starts to gather. How will I get in? I pull my phone from
my bag and dial the number of the contact I've been given.

'There are reporters and cameramen everywhere,' I
say. 'I don't know how to get in.'

A reassuring voice from the other end of the phone
tells me to stay where I am, they'll come and find me,
and a few moments later there's a smiling face, a hand
waving from the crowd.

'This way, Wendy!'

I follow her along the red carpet, my brogues unsuited to a walkway more used to celebrity heels, and now we're inside, away from the chaos outside. I breathe a sigh of relief and follow the young woman to meet the others. We meet inside the journalists' area and there's a buzz as reporters and TV presenters flit around us, rehearsing lines or deep in research notes preparing for their own meetings with the big star. I sit down with my new friends, also invited here by the Alzheimer's Society, mostly watching everything that's going on around us, commenting every few moments about how exciting it all is. I sip at my tea, clinging on to the sense of normality my cuppa offers me, the smile growing on my face as I become used to the surroundings. There's too much going on to decipher any conversation, so those of us with dementia are happy to sit quietly, just watching, having no expectation of conversation or filling in the blanks between us. And then at the windows we see a flash of light bulbs.

'This must be Julianne,' someone says, and I feel a flip inside.

She sweeps into the room in a beautiful black snakeskin-patterned dress, and is immediately descended on by reporters. While she does various interviews, I'm taken away to do my own for Radio 4's *Today* programme. When I return, the room has started to empty, the journalists, happy with the quotes they've got, have left to watch the film, and we have Julianne to ourselves. She is so refreshingly normal and unpretentious, chatting to each of us as though she's known us forever, remembering our names, making us feel special. She tells us many stories about the research she's done for the role, and we laugh and nod, knowing that a moment later all the anecdotes will be lost.

'You have the advantage over us,' I say. 'Because you'll remember our meeting, whereas we'll all forget.'

We laugh.

'Do you think I got the role right, Wendy?' Julianne asks.

'One thing you got spot on was the eyes,' I tell her. 'Your eyes told me you had dementia.'

And she smiled, happy to hear that.

'How do you live your life?' she asks.

'I live for the moment. I don't plan any more. I just enjoy each day as it comes.'

And as Julianne nods, for a moment I have that strange feeling again, as if Alzheimer's is a gift, as if we could all learn something from the harsh lessons it teaches.

She doesn't rush us and happily signs everything we've brought along, then she asks for a group photo as well as pictures with each of us individually. She says goodbye to each of us, remembering our names again, and then she's whisked away, back to her people.

That evening, at home, I watch a Channel 4 interview with Julianne Moore, and the reporter mentions my name to her. Her eyes light up and a smile spreads across her entire face.

'I've met Wendy!' she beams. 'Wendy is great! Wendy said that she used to plan a year in advance. She doesn't do that now – she plans the next week, she thinks about what's happening now and she's grateful for the present, and [that] she's alive. And, in a sense, that's how we all need to live our lives, really holding on to what we have, because that's the only thing we truly know about.'

There it is again, that sense of what Alzheimer's can give, not just take away.

A few days later, I wake in the morning to see emails and texts. Julianne Moore has won a leading actress BAFTA for her role in *Still Alice*. Not only that, but she mentioned me in her acceptance speech. It all feels quite surreal, a Hollywood star talking about me in front of the whole world. I cross the room, pick up the copy of the novel that Julianne signed for me and open the title page.

To Wendy, so happy to know you, with love and thanks, Julianne.

Two months later I am pacing some different London streets, walking back and forth between my hotel and the BBC studios to make sure that tomorrow morning I know where I'm going and what landmarks to look out for. I walk the route twice and return to my hotel with a sandwich and a drink before it gets dark. This big city feels unnerving and disorientating after hours, when the lights go down and others brighten up, when buildings are a ghostly shadow of their daylight selves. I prefer then to watch it from behind the safety of my hotel window. I am here to watch the camcorder recordings that I put together for the Victoria Derbyshire programme. They were originally meant to coincide with the release of *Still Alice*, but it needed to be put back a few weeks. After watching the recordings, we'll be interviewed in the studios, but the most exciting thing for me is the opportunity to meet Keith Oliver at last. It was, after all, his video on YouTube of life with dementia that had made me see this disease so differently, had made me believe there *is* a life after diagnosis, and what we were doing tomorrow will be living proof of that.

The following morning, I arrive at the BBC and find Katie from the Alzheimer's Society press office waiting with a smile in reception. There, too, is Keith and his wife Rosemary. I hug them both, already feeling that they are friends. There are a couple of other people with dementia there, and we're all shown to the green room, where I notice that their partners or children fuss around them, making sure they're comfortable, their coats are off and tidied, they've got a cup of tea. I notice that each of them has someone, but before I have time to dwell on that, or what it means to me, Katie presses a cup of hot tea in my hand, and my thoughts evaporate like steam.

We're taken down to the studio in turn, microphones are slipped under our clothes, and then Keith and I take our places on the sofa next to Jeremy Hughes, chief executive of the Alzheimer's Society. The floor manager counts down and we're on air.

'Over the next thirteen minutes you'll see an amazing film about living with dementia ...' Victoria says to the camera, and then I sit and watch alongside everyone else. I recorded hours of footage for Jim – not that I can remember any of it – but I knew what I had done would need to squeeze into just a few minutes. The film starts and I'm there again, back in the hospital corridor at work as I recreate that sense of disorientation; it takes me straight back to that moment, and I know if it makes me feel like that, audiences will understand better too. We watch Keith's video, see how he counts each of the items for his bathroom routine out of a basket and back in again, to be sure he's had a shave that morning. We see, too, how Christopher is at a stage in his disease where he can't remember the word for moon, but it doesn't matter, he knows it's something beautiful in the sky, isn't that enough? Do we really need to remember every single word as we go about our daily lives?

The interviews are over in seconds and while Keith and I agree live TV isn't exactly enjoyable, we know we're making a difference with everything we agree to do or be part of.

As we leave, Jim hands me two DVDs, one of the final recording and one of all of the hours of recordings I made. I know on there is a chat between myself, Gemma and Sarah around the kitchen table, and at some time in the future – who knows when – they will watch it and it will give them some comfort, a memory that has long escaped me.

I leave and head back home to Yorkshire, putting the experiences of the day down to another wonderful opportunity that has come my way thanks to my dementia diagnosis. There seems nothing wrong in making a list of the advantages of having Alzheimer's. Perhaps it might even help.

Do you remember your first day of work? I can still see you in that grey pinstripe suit, the smart white blouse underneath. You were thirty-nine then and that day felt like the first of the rest of your life. It was your best year yet. You weren't nervous walking through those automatic doors into the physiotherapy department, just excited. Inside was a packed waiting room, and there sat your new chair behind the reception desk. For the first morning you just watched what to do, and by the afternoon you were picking up phones. It made you feel so proud being able to answer and say: 'Physiotherapy, Wendy speaking, how can I help you?' I can't even use a phone now — it's too disorientating, people talk too fast — but you would chatter back, multitasking all the time, the phone crooked under your neck while you made an appointment on the computer, smiling at the next patient waiting at your desk. These things would be impossible for me, but they were nothing to you. The phone never stopped ringing, but it didn't faze you. You'd pride yourself on your memory, how you remembered the names of patients even months between appointments. Your colleagues were amazed, but you knew it added that personal touch, that it made patients feel special. Your memory was your thing, so you made it your mission to never forget.

The end, when it comes, is swift and sharp. I have never been one for long goodbyes, which is ironic, considering the disease that I have means I'm losing a little bit of me every day.

It is March 2015 and my last day at work. My team know I wouldn't want a fuss, so one of them hands over the cards and presents to me early in the morning, before anyone else arrives. I only stay in the office for two hours; anything more would be just too painful. I leave with a clipped goodbye, just as I did every evening, only this time I am not going to return. I don't leave that way because I don't care, but because perhaps I care too much.

I'm out in the corridor now, the cool air filling my lungs, and yet they still feel tight. I'm through one set of double doors and then the next, each step taking me further away from the twenty-year career I've loved. I'm numb inside, let down by a system that isn't willing to support people with dementia to stay at work, that can't adapt and change like those of us living with it do. I know that life will carry on without me, and I'm proud that my staff will manage, but I resent a management system that no longer needs me. My career had made me feel valued, but now I feel worthless.

I don't even try and remember this day. I don't want to. Perhaps that's why I have little to write here.

I'm not ready to say goodbye.

It was never a pleasant journey to the hospice in Halfpenny Lane, was it? You always felt sad driving into the car park, never knowing if this visit would be the last. How cruel the cancer was that had eaten away at your mother's body. It was different once you walked through the doors though, a daughter clinging to each hand. You noticed their grip was tighter than usual, unsure, uncertain. They took their cue from you and so you had to be strong. Inside, the hospice wasn't a depressing place, carrying an unspoken whisper that the patients inside deserved to die well, just as they had lived.

Your mother's room was at the end of a very dark corridor. Is that right or did it only feel that way? But once inside, her room looked out on to a beautiful garden filled with magnolia and cherry trees that, once bathed in the spring sunshine, would bud again with pretty pink blossom. Not that you knew if your mother would be there to see another season make its round. How differently we measure time when it is held inside the hands of a terminal illness. The cancer had spread quickly and her eye was the first to go. She missed little things, like being able to read a newspaper, and you coped as you always did, with practicality and resilience, taking her old spectacles to the opticians and convincing them to adapt them just for one eye. There was always a way — that's what you said. One day you arrived, the girls gave Nanna a quick hug, said hello, then ran off to the TV room, the dimmed sound of cartoons filtering back into the bedroom where you sat beside Mum. She was weak that day, the moments of lucidity coming and going.

'Tell me about school, Sarah,' she said, patting the bed beside her and trying a smile. 'What do you like doing best?'

You glanced over your shoulder, in case Sarah had appeared at the door, but no one was there and Mum stared expectantly at you. You could have corrected her, but her hazel eyes were alive for a second, in that glistening way that happens to grown-ups when they speak to children. You couldn't bear to dim the light from them and so you played along.

'It's good, Nanna,' you said, tentatively at first. But when she nodded, and reached for your hand, the smile reaching her eyes, you continued. 'I like painting and doing sums.'

'Have you played with your friends in the playground?' she asked.

'Yes,' you lied.

Then she looked straight past you and her face lit up in delight.

'Can you see that, Sarah?'

You followed her gaze but the room was still, nothing had come or gone, the only sign of life being the net curtains billowing at the windows.

'What can you see?' you asked.

'The soldiers,' she said, her face alive with nothing more than the thought. 'Coming over that hill, marching home from the war. Can you hear them singing?'

You couldn't bring yourself to break her heart. Why should you? What purpose would it have served? And so instead you played along, aiding and abetting the morphine. There was nothing else to do. Why confuse her further? you thought. And so you sat there together, watching the soldiers coming home, as Mum drifted back to sleep.

I wake quickly, wondering if I have missed my alarm, and then I remember, there's nothing to get up for. The clock beside my bedside stays silent these days. If I have a bad night's sleep and worry there are only a few short hours until the sun bleaches the black night blue, it doesn't matter. This is the life of the newly retired, and it takes some getting used to. I sink back into my pillow, but I'm distracted by the clock: 4.30 a.m. My body still used to the old schedule, dementia not yet overriding that internal alarm. Which day is it? I work it out slowly on my hands. Wednesday.

It had seemed when I first retired that there would be so many empty Wednesdays ahead; all the other days of the week, too. But that hasn't been the case. Today I'm grateful not to be heading far: a research event in Leeds, where I will be talking about the valuable work that Join Dementia Research is doing. It makes a change to travel somewhere relatively close by when all the other days since my last at work have been filled with trips far and wide: to Bradford University to help Ph.D. students, up to the West of Scotland University, speaking at an event and taking part in a social research study on employment after a diagnosis of dementia, back and forth to London for meetings with the Alzheimer's Society Research Network, or to speak at various events about my own diagnosis. Life is busier now, more varied and challenging than it ever was when I was at work, just in different ways.

It definitely hasn't been the emptiness of my weeks that has been difficult to get used to, but a certain loss inside. I couldn't put my finger on it at first, but then it came to me: all that information I kept ticking over inside my brain about work, all those rotas and staff, all those things-to-do lists, were now obsolete. It has been strange getting used to the space that has been left in this absence. But it has slowly been filled with the endless talks I've been invited to attend, the number of things that I learned about my disease, all helping me to under-stand it – and this new me – a little better. Research seems to be the way forward; every day I learn more and more about just how much people are trying to understand the disease. That's why I became a Join Dementia Research Champion, encouraging others to sign up to a new database that will match researchers with volunteers, or why I've offered to road test a new app for people with dementia, which has a variety of things to help with memory, including face recognition in case you forget who someone is. There's something else that motivates me, something a little more selfish: being involved in research means I'm contributing to changing the future for my daughters and generations beyond theirs, so that one day a diagnosis might not be filled with emptiness, but with hope of a cure and better understanding and conditions in care homes.

There are other little adjustments I've had to make in my retirement too, silly things like that great British pastime of checking the weather forecast. Before, I'd only ever checked whether it would be sunny on the weekend, but now if it's nice midweek I can sit outside in my garden, watching the birds as they flit between feeders.

I feel my stomach rumble, a sensation I was never used to before in the mornings when I had little time to get myself showered and dressed and on the bus by 5.30 a.m. Now there is time to eat a slice of toast or some porridge with a cup of tea in the morning, and so my body sets an internal alarm, and it's already thinking about lunch before I've finished wiping the crumbs away.

Colleagues had said: 'You'll have so much time when you retire,' but that hasn't been the case yet. Instead I wonder how I ever had the time to work. I settle back into my pillow, pulling the duvet up to my chin. There are a few more hours to doze before I need to get up and get on.

***

Do you remember visiting someone with dementia once, long before your own diagnosis? You often went to wards as part of your job. You were seeing staff mostly, but one day you lingered longer on a ward for the elderly. The nursing staff were moaning about one particular patient with dementia who was causing chaos and wouldn't settle down. You spotted him, sitting in the corner with worry in his eyes. He was clearly agitated, asking anyone who would listen where his wife was. The conversation with the nurses melted into background noise, and you found yourself walking over to him, taking up a seat beside his. You started talking to him.

'Where do you think your wife might be?' you asked, gently.

'I don't know,' he said, anxiety biting at his lips. It was all he could do not to break down.

So you asked him about her, and as he talked, a light went on in his blue eyes. They started to twinkle again, and he smiled as — just for a second — she was brought back to life by his imagination. You asked to see a photo, but he didn't have one to show. Perhaps that was why he gabbled on about her? He had no way of 'seeing' his wife, except in images conjured up in his heart. So you suggested to the nurses that the family bring in a photograph of her. It turned out she'd been dead a while, but he didn't remember. Or at least not in that moment. Any talk of her passing, of people reminding him she was dead, just sent him into a spin, mourning her passing once again. So why not let him look at her? Why not let her keep him company once again in the evening of his life in amongst the trays of hospital food, the vases of wilting flowers and card games started and never finished?

The next time you went back to the ward, he had a photograph on his bedside table. He didn't remember you, and that was OK. When you asked who the lovely lady was in the photo, his face broke into the biggest smile, as he spoke so proudly of his wife, beginning her story again, bringing her back to life. He'd forget that she never visited, and whenever he did ask the nurses where she was, they distracted him, asking questions about her. And then he was content again. She was real.

It would have been cruel to keep telling that man that his beloved wife was dead. If he didn't remember, she wasn't dead to him.

I shoot up in bed. My skin is clammy. I blink and see it again: the nightmare that had crept into my dreams. It has been happening a lot recently, a frightening picture pulling me to consciousness, bizarre and terrible things – the other day it was bears running along with buckets of blood. I check the clock: 3 a.m. I know I won't sleep for the rest of the night. This is my life now, no more than a few hours of snatched sleep. In the day I'm exhausted and plagued by headaches. I know I used to sleep solidly, waking only when the alarm went off, but now it can take me hours to get to sleep, staring at the outside world through a gap in the curtains. I close my eyelids, but my eyes are awake behind them, darting back and forth. If I sleep, it's for an hour or so, and then so lightly it feels as if I wake in the middle of dreams.

I open my laptop and search 'sleep deprivation and dementia': thousands of results come up but nothing that explains why. I decide instead to write a blog about it, hoping that the world outside my curtains might offer up an explanation.

The following morning, I wake to dozens of replies, many asking whether I am currently taking donepezil, a drug introduced ten years ago and believed to slow the progression of Alzheimer's. When I'd started taking it a year ago, I'd been so hopeful that it would give me extra time with my daughters. But at 3 a.m., longing for sleep when your time on earth ticks by in long seconds, the advantages of a so-called wonder drug pales in comparison to the side effects. Someone suggests taking it in the morning instead of the recommended night-time dose.

The first night of taking it in the morning, I knew that my head felt calmer and that night was the first night in two years that I hadn't had disturbing dreams, one lady had written. *The first night I hadn't woken and frantically had to work out what was real and what had been a dream.*

I decide to follow her advice, and that night I have my first sleep free of nightmares – still not the whole way through, but much better. I'm pleased for another reason: I don't want to stop taking donepezil. It's always been considered a drug that is given to reduce or manage the symptoms of those of us with mild to moderate Alzheimer's, but a recent study found that withdrawing the drug from people living with the disease doubled the chances of them being moved into a nursing home after a year. It seems that the drug keeps on working much longer than anyone originally thought, and with the annual cost of care homes being in the tens of thousands, and the annual cost of donepezil being just over £20, I know which one makes more sense. I want to be able to stay in my home for as long as possible and so the scales tip back the other way, and I can happily give up a perfect night's sleep for another year at home.

There is something special about wandering around York in the rain. I am walking along the famous Shambles in the drizzle, the cobbled streets shiny from the showers, the timber-framed shops, hundreds of years old, leaning over in that higgledy-piggledy fashion, so close that I'm surprised they don't touch the sides of my red umbrella. This street has long since stopped selling the meat it was once famous for, but the butchers' slabs remain outside shop windows, filled with tourists in the summer, who stop and lean on them while reaching into their bags for cold drinks. Not today though, everyone else is sheltering from the rain, so the streets are fairly empty as I shuffle through them. These are well-trodden steps and I'm used to navigating the cobbles, especially with fewer tourists to get in the way of my wobbling gait. At the end of the street I turn right into Kings Square, where a street entertainer plays to a bedraggled crowd, who are doing a good job of ignoring the downpour while wet hair sticks to their faces and water swells at their feet.

I stand for a few moments, smiling to myself. Only, when I look up again, the place where I was standing has gone. I spin around, scanning the buildings, but nothing is familiar. The trees whizz by, red-brick buildings and small Georgian panelled windows, but no clues. Where am I? I look at the people close by, but blank faces stare back, strangers. Panic rises then; it comes from deep inside my chest, stealing the breath from me as it does. I try to take deep breaths, but they're too fast, too sudden, my head feels light. Where to go? The busker still sings and it's too loud, each twang of his guitar stripping thoughts from my mind. I'm scared. I'm lost.

I stumble back through the crowd, looking for an open space, staggering this way and that. Lanes shoot off from the square, odd-shaped streets with strange pebbly floors that mean nothing to me. Now I'm frozen to the spot, too scared to move. My eyes scan, searching for something familiar, a clue. *How did I get here? Where had I come from?* The rain: I need to get inside. I see a café sign then, over the heads of people in the crowd, blue and familiar; something draws me to the safety of it. I cross the square. A car beeps its horn. I jump, but carry on across the road. I need to get inside, to think and sit, and wait for the fog to lift. How did it descend so quickly? Like driving on a bright day right into a thick cloud.

I go into the café, find a seat in the corner and sit. Droplets of water drip into my shoes. I'm still. I don't register the other faces or look at the staff. I know I'll be safe here, an instinct breaking through the mist. I stare out of the window, the scene beyond it still alien. *Look away*, I tell myself. Instead I reach for my red haversack and pull a newspaper from it. I flick through the pages, my eyes scanning the black and white, not taking in any of the words or stories or pictures, just waiting. Waiting for the world to clear. Waiting for time to pass. How long do I sit there before a sound cuts through? The busker playing outside. I look out of the window and there he is. And beyond him, a familiar chocolate shop; next to that, a biscuit shop, the baker's on the corner; the square is coming back into focus. I manage a smile.

I sit there a little while longer, just to be sure. I get a coffee and stare out at the square I know so well but which had been lost in an instant. How did that happen? A short circuit in my brain, a disconnect somewhere between my eyes. I'm reminded that this disease can steal the past, the present and the future.

The sun has broken through the clouds by the time I leave. I shuffle back through familiar streets to home.

***

None of us are born with fear: it accumulates alongside life experiences, and I can still remember where your fear of animals came from. It sounds ridiculous now, but you never had pets, so the idea was alien to you. When you were a child, you were chased one day on your scooter by a large black dog, barking and baring its teeth. The fear you felt was enough to see you through the rest of your life. After that you'd cross the road to avoid someone walking a dog and cats were the same — the hairs on the back of your neck would curl up if you passed one sitting happily on a garden wall. When Gemma got cats you were terrified of all of them, so much so that she'd put them out whenever you went round to her house.

Billy, a handsome black cat with yellow-green eyes, made you very wary. If he walked into the room while you were there, you were instantly nervous and on edge. It was as if he knew, as if they all knew — they gave you a wide berth, too. Was it mutual dislike or respect? It didn't matter as long as they weren't near. How different you are from me; if only I'd been there to act as a conduit. Just the other day I was looking after Billy for Gemma; each time I do, I'm sure that he can hear my stick and shuffle coming round the corner of the house, because I put my key in the front door and he's sitting waiting for me every single time. You probably would have refused to cross the threshold when you spotted those two big eyes staring up at you, anxiety would start eating away inside, but for me all stress dissolves at the sight of him.

Billy pads into the kitchen, performing a tiny dance in front of my feet before he finds the patch of sunshine on the kitchen tiles. He flops down on to it while I scratch the back of his ears and he purrs his approval. I shake some biscuits into his bowl and he gets up and crunches on them noisily. He's only allowed a few, as Gemma has put him on a diet. She's not sure why he's put on so much weight recently; even the vet commented on it.

I make myself a cup of tea, and as the kettle boils I feel Billy's tail curling around my legs. I glance at his empty bowl.

'Oh Billy, have I forgotten to feed you?'

He looks up with big, sad eyes, his purr audible over the boiling kettle that switches itself off. I shake a few biscuits into his bowl.

I know our routine after this, despite the fact that so many other things desert my memory every single day. I sit and sip my tea, and he paces around looking for the piece of red string with slivers of gold, the one I used to decorate his Christmas gift. It has become his favourite toy. He disappears and I find him on the stairs, sitting beside it, saying, 'Here it is,' with those yellow-green eyes. We go up to the loft room – more space to play there – and I tie a knot in the end for him to catch in his claws and our game continues until he loses interest. Afterwards, I sit down in the chair. Billy comes to sit beside me, and as we look out over the orchard, just to have him near makes me feel calm inside. He jumps up on to my lap and I run my fingers through his soft fur.

I know I wouldn't have been able to do this before, but I've learned so much from animals. This change in my personality, this softening in one part of my brain, has meant that I've made time to sit and stop and watch, much like they do. Animals lead a simple life — they live in the moment, and that's what I've found I have in common with Billy, an appreciation of now. Many fears have left me now. Perhaps it's because nothing can be more frightening than dementia. I live every day with the unknown, which is possibly why I'm not afraid any more: of cats, of the dark, of the disease.

A few moments later we hear the front door open, and both of us go downstairs to greet Gemma home from work. We meet her in the kitchen, flick on the kettle for a cup of tea and while Billy sits on my lap, Gemma and I catch up on the day. Twenty minutes must pass like that and then Billy jumps down from my lap and sniffs at his empty bowl, then sits staring at it.

'Ooh,' I say. 'I must have forgotten.'

Gemma looks at him, unsure. 'The vet said Billy has to lose weight, but he must be getting fed by someone else, because his diet isn't working. You are only giving him a few biscuits when you're on Billy duty, aren't you, Mum?'

'Oh yes, I'm sure I do,' as I shake more biscuits into his bowl and Billy purrs happily.

I'm sitting in front of the consultant while he scribbles down the results of my latest set of mini memory tests. From the other side of his desk, I try and fail to read his writing. Finally, he sits back and sighs.

'You're a little worse than last time,' he says, and despite the fact I know I have a progressive illness, I feel my heart sink inside my chest.

I shuffle out of his office, feeling sad that my diseased brain has let me down yet again. I don't know exactly how or where, on which part of the test or which specific questions. All I can remember is the word 'worse'. I go to sleep with the word 'worse' settling down on the pillow with me.

Of course I know I won't get better, but I often think now about how important the doctor's choice of words and use of language is when speaking to patients. Might I have felt less helpless if he'd said: 'This time you scored twenty-six; it seems your coordination was the problem. What can we do to help with that?'

Just leaving out the negative word 'worse' would give hope that I could find some way to outwit the part of my brain that is no longer working as it should. It would also give me some confidence in the bits that are still working well, and perhaps even some insight – for example, my game of Scrabble every morning seems to be helping, so I'll keep doing that. I would feel empowered, rather than helpless. I could help myself.

Like other people, when I was given my diagnosis I was told: 'There's nothing we can do, I'm afraid.' I can still remember the feelings of loss and fear and hopelessness, and in the days and weeks that followed, all I could think of was that word 'afraid'. It felt so negative, so scary. They were 'afraid' there was nothing they could do. I was 'afraid' there was nothing they could do. What about if instead I'd been told in a different way: 'Yes, the diagnosis is dementia. I'll put you in touch with people who can help you to adapt, people who also have a diagnosis so you can share tips and tricks.' Immediately I would have had hope.

A few weeks later I'm standing in front of a group of student nurses as I deliver a talk. They sit eagerly in front of me, their hands in their laps, guarding notebooks and pens, and I start by asking them which words spring to mind when they hear the word 'dementia'. I turn to the whiteboard as they call them out: *Demented, senile, burden, sufferer, old age, living death* …

I pause and look out at the room.

'Imagine how that makes me feel to hear you say such words,' I say. 'I mean, I know I look old and my hair is a bit grey, but that's because I don't dye it – unlike your lecturer, Rob!'

He pretends to squirm and everyone laughs.

'But in the grand scheme of things, I'm relatively young to have developed dementia. And do I look like I'm "suffering"? Do I seem to be a "burden"?'

I hear a few pairs of feet shuffle uncomfortably. I write down the words on the white board and then turn back to them to explain how positive language leads to positive well-being and how negative language brings anyone down.

'If your boss were to tell you day after day that you were stupid, it would bring you down and you'd start to believe it,' I say. 'That's how we feel when you continually tell us we're "suffering" from dementia. A diagnosis of dementia is bad enough – that's devastating news – but that's where negative language can stop and positive language can begin. If someone tells you day after day that you are a sufferer, you end up believing it. We "struggle" on a daily basis to outmanoeuvre the challenges we face but, often with help, we can find ways of overcoming those struggles.'

I have the full attention of everyone in the room. I tell them they can replace the word 'suffering' with 'living with'.

'I'm not denying or minimising the considerable challenges we face. I'm simply saying it sounds better,' I say. And they nod. They're getting it too.

I think back to my own diagnosis, and how it was only actively changing my point of view that replaced impossible with possible. 'I like to concentrate on what I can do, not what I can't do, but sometimes we need your help to do this.'

I tell them how the media don't help either, always referring to 'dementia sufferers', and how dispiriting the images are, too, such as the photographs of bed-bound old ladies that I'd found when I'd first googled dementia. I tell them about the support groups I've sat in, the husbands who bring their wives, or vice versa, and how the partner always speaks for them, describing their wife as 'suffering' from dementia. How, when it gets to my turn, I always say: 'I'm not suffering, I'm *living with* dementia.' I tell them about the one time I did that and how the wife who was being spoken for lifted her gaze to meet mine, the seed sown in her head; dementia didn't have to be the end. It wasn't for me.

There have been many moments over the last few months when I've felt the empty space by my side where a significant other should be. There is a picture that exists in the back of our minds of spending the evening of our life with someone else to keep a watch over us. We know our children will have lives and families of their own, but we never picture ourselves alone. I would be lying if I didn't say that there have been moments when I've looked around a room and missed having someone with me. At the *Still Alice* premiere, everyone seemed to be in couples. Everyone with dementia there had their own walking memory beside them who could make sure they'd taken their tablets, or eaten, or had a drink that day. But there is another side of me who has seen the pain that's written across the faces of loved ones who watch their partners decline. I have often thought that I wouldn't like the pressure of a husband for that reason.

There are other things too. When you live with some-one it's quite natural to move things around, to tidy up or to be messy, but all of those things would be unhelpful to me. I used to be really tidy, but now I leave paperwork out, because if I put it away out of sight it stops existing for me. My kitchen worktops are strewn with papers that I need to let me know what I'm doing for the week ahead: the conferences where I'm giving talks, the places in London or elsewhere in the UK I need to go to meet with a research committee or a steering group. Now I am the messy one. If I lived with someone messy and things were in my way that wouldn't normally be there, I'd constantly be tripping over. It's true I don't have someone to jog my memory, someone to be a back-up brain or a constant companion, someone to laugh with or just to hug me when things go wrong. But I also don't have to worry if I've upset someone by not remembering something, or someone urging me to eat when I'm not hungry, correcting me, finishing my sentences, or fussing when I'm having a bad day.

Yes, the picture in my head looks a little different from the one I might have imagined for my retirement, but my independent nature – which has so far defeated this disease – would never want someone to take over tasks just because they're taking me a little longer.

So perhaps that space by me is there for a reason.

You were sitting on the little wall outside the back door, mug of tea in hand, staring out at the summer flowers that had broken through the soil. Being a single mum was still very new and some days were lonelier than others. A voice snapped you out of your thoughts.

'Fancy bringing your cuppa over here?' You looked up and saw Julie's cheery smile peering through the gap in the fence. Her husband Terry had taken a fence panel out months ago so the children could move between the two back gardens – her two boys and your two girls. Altogether you made a nice big family, and that's still what you needed to feel some days, part of a family. Julie and Terry Feegrade weren't without their own problems. Their eldest son, Jason, hadn't been expected to survive more than a few years, and even now he couldn't speak or hear.

You signed 'hello' to him, sitting happily in his wheelchair, as you went through the fence with your cup of tea.

I wonder if the Feegrades ever realised just how much they meant to you and the girls. There were Christmases they wouldn't hear of you spending on your own, always making an extra three seats at their table for you. Everyone would budge up, elbows knocking each other as you tucked into a roast turkey dinner, and Julie's infamous curry was always there for anyone wanting an alternative. It just made it more fun to be all together. There was the time you all went on holiday to Spain – the girls would have been about seven and four then – and the three of you were more excited about a first ride in an aeroplane than anything else. You'd landed in the pitch black and then Terry had handed you the keys to a hire car.

'We've got two cars,' he'd said. 'And no one else can drive apart from me and you.'

There wasn't any time for nerves, so you got behind the wheel in the dead of night and followed him on the wrong side of the road to the villa you'd hired between you. You'd gripped the steering wheel all the way, terrified, but by the time you stepped out of the car and hauled the suitcases from the boot, you were thrilled by the challenge.

You'd even taught Julie to drive once you were back in the UK, your lessons filled with danger and near misses, but most of all laughter. There was the time when you persuaded her to try and overtake a milk float on the dual carriageway; she'd gone into second gear instead of fourth and lost her confidence, so you'd both sat giggling as you trundled along at 20 mph.

Those were the friends who filled the gap where someone else should have been, who laughed and listened, who fetched tissues and made tea when you cried. Who made life fun for the girls on the days when the world seemed to cave in on you, and just like that, day by day, you got through it and came out the other side. Stronger. Better. Happier. Because friends were everything.

When you moved to York you found a teabag one Christmas in the shops that perfectly summed up your relationship with Julie. It had a little tag on it that read: I cannot sit and chat with you, just like we used to do, so make yourself a cup of tea, I'll think of you, you think of me.

I'm outside in the front garden, pulling weeds from where they hide under stones, when I see him, my neighbour, Jim, walking down the street as usual. I wait for him to walk right by my house. I drop the fork from my hand and push myself up on my knees, ready to greet him with a smile, but as I do he crosses the road to walk on the other side. I look back to the soil for a second, confused. This also happened yesterday, and the day before that. He'd normally pass with a cheery smile and wave, or he'd stop and we'd comment on the weather in that terribly British way. But for the last few days, nothing, and yesterday, I knew he'd seen me.

I'm about to start picking at a few stray green strands left in the soil when it hits me: the article that I'd done for the local newspaper a few days before, explaining that I had been diagnosed with dementia and all the work I've been doing since to raise awareness. Jim reads that paper. Could this be why he's avoiding me? I need to know. I stand up and brush the last of the soil from my trousers, then I'm out of the garden gate, crossing the road towards him.

'Jim?' I call.

He puts his head down, sure that he's about to walk past straight past me, but instead I say hello in my cheeriest way.

He mumbles hello back, but doesn't seem keen to stop and chat.

'Have I done something to offend you?' I ask, puzzled.

He stops then. His eyes flick away, keen to avoid my own.

'I-I saw you in the local paper,' he says.

I laugh. 'Fame at last! Although they could have taken a better photograph and made me look ten years younger!' He looks uncomfortable. 'Is that the reason you're not speaking to me?'

He sighs. 'I just didn't know what to say.'

'The picture wasn't that bad, was it?' I laugh, trying to lighten the mood.

He looks down at his feet on the pavement and shuffles his weight. I don't mean to embarrass him.

'How can you have dementia when you ride your pink bicycle?' he asks.

This time I don't make light of it. I can see that he doesn't understand, so I start at the beginning.

'Dementia has to start somewhere,' I explain. 'It doesn't always mean the end stages, and I'm just an example of someone at the start of the journey. I'm no different from the day before you saw the article; we were chatting that day.'

He nods, as if it's sinking in slowly, somewhere. He goes off for his newspaper, his gait a little slower this time, more thoughtful.

But the next morning when he passes by the house, he doesn't cross the road. In fact, he walks right up, newspaper under his arm, and we chat about all sorts — especially the weather.

'Are you OK?' he asks, a little more carefully than he has before.

'Yes, thank you,' I tell him with a smile.

He goes on his way, satisfied.

If only it were that easy to explain to everyone, because I have noticed that more than just a few friends have gone to ground since they heard about my diagnosis, some who I have known my entire life, and it has been hurtful. There have been the emails sent that have never received a reply; at first I put it down to busy lives and eventually send another. Again, into the ether. There have been the friends who would make a point of getting in touch every couple of months, then I realised there had been silence. There were fewer Christmas or birth-day cards, less news travelling up and down the phone and broadband wires. People who had shared a lifetime with me now didn't seem to want to share a text or email. It wasn't something I noticed all of a sudden – it was a realisation that crept up on me. Where had every-one gone?

For every friend who had disappeared, there were, though, the ones who stayed, and they were full of empathy and love, and even practical solutions. The Feegrades, who read on my blog how often I woke up without a clue which day of the week it was, gave me a gift when I went to stay, a big bold bedside clock that had the day, month and year on it as well as the time.

I'd added the name of my blog on to my email signa-ture, so even if people weren't answering my emails, it was still possible to see what I was up to, even if their own news wasn't returned in the same way it once was. It took almost eighteen months for one very close friend to get back in touch. He asked if he could come over and take me out for supper, and when he saw that I could still string a sentence together, I watched as his shoulders relaxed away from his ears. He's never mentioned the word 'dementia' to me – not even now – but at least he's back in touch.

Another two friends admitted they'd followed my blog, even if they hadn't been in touch with me directly.

We felt so stupid for thinking that you'd be anything other than positive and still active, they wrote when they decided to get in touch again.

But I was still me. Still me, but with a diseased brain. What is it about this kind of illness that makes people so frightened? Is it the thought that it might happen to them? Is it rubbing shoulders with their own mortality that scares them away? What do I remind them of, or make them fear? Is it simply the future, because my own brain is only declining the way everyone else's does eventually, but at ten times the speed? But they can't discover the truth about dementia unless I welcome them back in, which I do. I have to. There is no point in educating strangers if I can't make even those closest to me understand. Just like Jim, they'd heard a diagnosis of Alzheimer's and pictured me in a care-home bed, waiting to die. But could I blame them when that had been the exact same image over-whelming my own brain back at the beginning?

It was my words that changed everything, but not spoken ones, written ones. Dementia may have stolen the words from my mouth, it might have made it harder for me to grasp hold of the ones I'm searching for in time to finish a sentence, but the part of my brain that can type fluently is still intact. Friends are amazed when they read how I spend my days going up and down the country attending conferences and overseeing clinical trials, then writing all my findings down in my blog so I can help others.

'You're busier now than you were when you were working,' more than one has said, and it is true.

I'm keeping myself busy now to forget the fact that I'm losing the past. I'm creating memories and keeping them safe on my blog so I can hang on to the present, and create a new type of personal history, simply because I don't know what the future holds. But friends and family are the keepers of the past, they are the guardians of the bits that dementia can't steal. They may not have the exact same memory that I do of events, but they were there, they can tell me, or they can listen while I tell them, so it seems more important than ever to hold on to the people who bore witness to my life. They will, after all, be best placed to tell me what it was like once dementia has done its work.

There is another benefit to being friends with me of course: they can talk to me, pour out the most confident details of their lives and I always remind them: 'Your secret is safe with me – I'll have forgotten by the time we walk out of the room.'

You loved the hustle and bustle of a city. The continual sirens weaving through the city walls and stationary traffic, the world alive with noise, every sound a clue to the vibrant environment surrounding you. It made you feel alive to be a part of that. You'd eavesdrop on tourists ambling through the cobbled streets of the Shambles, listening to their conversations and chatter, smiling or laughing at glimpses of their lives caught up among the chaos of the day. You liked the fact that the streets were busy, that you were one of a swarm of people making your way through the lanes. You liked the bikes that weaved around you as you crossed the road, the cars that beeped, waking up the tourists sleepwalking across the road or the ones staring up at the spires and steeples of York Minster. You liked being a part of that busy community, the way that every single one of your senses was stirred and stimulated by the buzz of life going on every time you stepped out of your front door. City life was the only life; you couldn't imagine being anywhere else. How alien all that seems to me now.

***

I walk out of my front door and it's there. It comes at me from every direction. It doesn't just hit my ears – it smashes into them, rolling around inside my brain. I swallow and down it goes, rumbling around inside my tummy. Noise is everywhere and much louder than before. I hadn't noticed it up until now, but more recently I've found myself cowering once I step outside the front door, as if the world has turned up its volume overnight without telling me. How I wish I could just reach for a remote control and turn it down again.

I walk outside my gate and press the button on the pedestrian crossing. The traffic lights turn red and the green man starts to flash as I cross the road, and I wince as I do, the beeps ringing in my ears louder and louder, a shrill sound that penetrates deep inside. I reach up and cover my ears with my hands; perhaps the council have adjusted the sound on the speaker, perhaps they really have made it louder while I slept? I carry on walking, but there is soon something else. In the distance I spot a flash of blue lights. I stop on the pavement, stepping back from the kerb in time to watch the ambulance go by, but when it races past I jump back a few feet, the noise taking my breath away, the sound still stinging inside long after the ambulance has disappeared up the road on its emergency mission. Why does noise suddenly hurt so much?

By the time I arrive home I am grateful for the peace it brings. I sit down in front of my computer and type 'heightened hearing and dementia' into the search bar, and I'm surprised by the number of results that spring up. I read page after page about other people who have experienced the world as a louder place since being diagnosed with dementia – all from those living with the disease, no explanations from medics. The more I read, the more my heart sinks into my lap. I sit back in my chair and I already know what this means: I'm going to have to leave my beloved city. I look around the walls of the house that I had been so sure would be my forever home, and I know that I will soon need to take pictures down from hooks and pack books into boxes. What was once my peaceful oasis, my calm in the middle of a busy city centre, is everything I don't need now. It is simply too noisy.

Over the next few days the sirens dashing through York seem to get louder and louder, though perhaps I'm just noticing them more. Our narrow streets weren't built to allow four-tonne ambulances through, and while they slow to navigate cobbled streets and centuries-old walls, I stop and cover my ears, pain penetrating my eardrums. The chatter of tourists is overwhelming, snippets of conversations now feeling like a swarm of bees inside my mind, making me lose track of my thoughts. A child's cry is so harsh and piercing it stops me still in the street. Everything that was part of the reason I loved the place, that made up a soundtrack rich with tones and tales of the city, is now the same reason I need to leave.

But where to go? Everything that I have read about dementia tells me that moving home after a diagnosis can be very unsettling, and so I push that thought to the back of my mind. Instead I buy earplugs, foam ones that mould themselves to the shape of my ear. I step outside and the world is a silent place; it reminds me of winter, when snow falls and lines the streets like cotton wool, muffling the sounds underneath with a thick blanket of fluffy white. But the earplugs take away something else – my ability to hear the sounds that are important, like the cyclist approaching from my right whose path I step into, almost knocking him off. I pull the plugs out apologetically, trying to explain. These are no good; I need something that will take the edge off but still allow me to hear some things. I find some bright-pink earplugs in a shop a few days later, and they do help, but they're not enough. The weeks go on as York slowly turns up the pitch, and then it seems impossible to ignore it any longer, to block out the sound. It's not York; it's me who has changed.

I start scouring the internet, looking for houses in quieter areas of York, but all of them are outside my budget. Without a job, I need money left over from the sale of my house to adapt a new home, to future-proof for whatever dementia has to throw at me. Day after day I give up on property searches, a heavy black feeling sitting deep inside my stomach as I close my laptop. I'm not ready for this change. I didn't ask for this to happen to me. I resent dementia for stealing the image of my future that I'd so carefully created in my head, as if the disease has just reached in there and plucked it out without me noticing. And all I can do is adapt.

This weekend I'm staying with Gemma and her boyfriend Stuart in their quiet little village 30 miles from York. I am settled in their spare room, having a moment's peace from the conversations over the TV downstairs. I stay in the converted loft room when I'm here, Billy often curled up in my lap, and I look out at the birds and nature, trees gently swaying in the breeze on the other side of the window, the only noise being the leaves rustling, or a faint tweet from a starling or thrush. Nothing too testing. I amuse myself in the daytime walking down to the village shop for a weekend newspaper, smiling and exchanging hellos with everyone that passes by. The people in the shop are so friendly. I always get the impression they know a little of everyone's life, and perhaps that's how places like this cling on to communities, by sharing little titbits. They haven't yet firmly closed their front doors, all life taking place behind net curtains. It can make a person feel safe.

And then I have an idea. I lift Billy off my knees and find my laptop to start searching for properties in the village. Could I be happy here on my own if Gemma ever moved away, I wonder, as a list of properties outside my price range pops up. I sigh, defeated, and close the laptop again, that sense of not belonging sitting awkwardly inside. Hadn't everything been mapped out before? Didn't I know where I was going – even where I'd been? Instead I'm left with blanks.

Over the next few weeks, I make more visits to the village, always with the same thought in my mind: could I be happy here? I notice more and more the tranquillity of the place. I stand beside the duck pond on the little decked path, throwing in special food sold at the village shop in tiny bags. Even the ducks are looked after here, and I sense they know they'll get more than their fair share from me, just like Billy does. I start seeing more benefits: the shop, the post office, the bus that goes straight into York from the town nearby. I wouldn't be giving up the city completely; it would still be there, at the end of the line.

I return to York a few days later and Sarah comes over to help me clear out some cupboards. The move will start before I've even found my home, I decide. There will be no last-minute packing this time, everything will need to be pared down months in advance. We start in the kitchen, getting rid of old cans of food or spices long past their sell-by date. I look twice at the date on the cans before I throw them away – that would never have happened before. We chat as we go, remembering stories from the numerous moves over the years. I start on a cupboard packed with kitchen utensils.

'Do you remember the garden at Hyde Close?' I ask, pulling a cheese grater from the cupboard.

'You would never imagine there had been a lawn under there,' Sarah says, remembering how it had taken me a whole week to cut back all that overgrowth.

I pull another cheese grater from the cupboard.

'And the state of those windows there! You and Gemma had to clean them with tiny toothbrushes, do you remember?'

I find another cheese grater, and put it in the pile, giving it a quizzical look as I do.

We carry on chatting as I go further back in the cupboard; there are ladles, wooden spoons, an apple corer. And another cheese grater.

'Strange,' I say, turning to the pile behind me. 'I've already found three of these.'

Sarah and I start laughing, but by the time we've reached the back of the cupboard, ten cheese graters line the kitchen worktop. We stare at them, both of us wondering how at some time I must have convinced myself I didn't have one.

'The strangest thing is, I don't even like cheese that much,' I say. 'Let alone grated cheese.'

We're giggling as we put together a bag to go to charity — nine cheese graters making up the bulk of it. It doesn't feel so bad then, thinking of the move, not with

Sarah beside me, laughing with me. I can do this. Just as soon as I find the right place.

Most people dread moving home, but you always saw it as a chance to have a clear-out, a chance to put old things in new places, to start again. You'd collect boxes for weeks before from the supermarket, you'd sit with your feet up long after the girls had gone to bed and make lists of all the things you needed to do. When it came to packing, you were a pro: brown parcel tape to seal the boxes, one room at a time systematically packed, a clue inked in black marker pen on each side of the box to tell you. Right-hand side of desk *was enough, your brilliant memory itemising everything that was there. Box after box was sealed and stacked neatly in the corner of the room, key items like hammers and screwdrivers, kettle and teabags all in the box labelled* Important Box *– the last to be Sellotaped up, the first to be opened the other end.*

You never told the girls until everything had been signed on the dotted line, just in case it all went wrong. The first time you moved it could have been sad, moving from the family home to a smaller house in Hyde Close, a quiet cul-de-sac just round the corner, but you made it exciting with tales of a better sweet shop nearby with a much broader selection than their current favourites. The new house had two double bedrooms and a small box room. It could have been a problem, but you knew Gemma liked all things tiny and you already had ideas about how to make it the perfect space, so by the time Sarah had claimed the bigger room, Gemma was sold. You noticed the little box room had a door that opened inwards when you looked around, and made a mental note to put the screwdriver in the 'important' box to remove it the minute you moved in.

On moving day the girls sat in the back of the car behind you, Important Box between them, chattering about the adventures you were going to have in the new house. You probably didn't hear them, too focused on the list in your pocket that you'd drawn up, the one detailing all the chores you needed to get on with in turn; cupboards to clean, paintwork to wipe, carpets to hoover. Each item waiting patiently to be crossed off.

As the removal men arrived, the girls zipped between empty rooms and up and down stairs, while you got to know the house yourself, peering through dusty windows at an overgrown garden you couldn't wait to get your secateurs on. But it would have to wait. As each box arrived, the girls looked hopefully for their treasures among them, every bit of organisation you'd put in at the other end making it easier for the removal men to do their job.

You'd look around at all the unpacking that needed to be done and would always start with the Important Box. Kettle on, teabags fished from the bottom and plonked in a mug, your ceremonial first cup of tea in the new house and squash made in familiar plastic tumblers. After that it didn't take too long to get everything straight. The girls were desperate to help, so you fished toothbrushes and Jif from Important Box. They looked up at you, confused at first, until you showed them the windows *in the bedroom and the black that had collected in the corners. Tiny hands for tiny jobs, They looked amazed when they saw how clean the toothbrush made it, and within moments the chatter was replaced by intense concentration, each trying her hardest to make her window the best. While they did that, you cleaned cupboards and vacuumed floors, wiped paintwork and made beds. The list got shorter and shorter and your satisfaction grew as you turned it black by scribbling things off.*

By the evening — the biggest boxes unpacked, the television tuned in, takeaway ordered as a special treat — it was feeling more like home already. Two days later it would look like you'd been there years. Then you remembered one more thing before putting your feet up: the door that needed to come off Gemma's room. Screwdriver retrieved, you climbed the stairs.

It happened again the other day. My diseased mind was playing tricks on me. I looked up in the half-light at Gemma's house and there was my mum bustling about in the hallway just how I remembered her; she was wearing the same long, multicoloured dress she always did, her two hip replacements never righting that limp. I sat perfectly still, remembering not to panic, while my eyes fought with my logical mind, raking through questions about dates and attempting maths to prove whether what was in front of me was as real as it looked. *What year are we in? Is she still alive? How old is Gemma? Does that give me any clues?* Mum turned to me and smiled then and in that moment I didn't feel afraid, just calm, confident even, as if I knew this wasn't real, more like I was being granted a gift, another chance to see her as she was. That my disease, and everything so terrible that it steals from me, had also allowed me a much-loved glimpse of the past.

Another time it had been Dad I'd seen, in the same half-light, but this time in my new house. He was never without a suit or jacket, except when he was relaxing at home, but this time he wore a cardigan, and I knew then he must feel at home in my new place. But he wore something else: the sadness that never left him after Mum's death. Just like Mum, he smiled and I smiled back, even though logic was trying so desperately hard to kick in and remind me that the man in front of me – so real to me – was nothing more than a trick of my mind.

Did I think in that moment that Mum and Dad were still alive? Probably. Did it really matter? Probably not. I don't need to be told over and over that Mum and Dad are dead; what difference does my fantasy make to anyone else? People without memory problems often forget that those of us with dementia think about things in the past, and so the helpful response is probably to 'go along' with our experience, rather than trying to pull us back into the present day. It's not unethical to do that; it's just valuing the person's experience, because for them, it's as real as this book you are holding in your hands right now.

I'm glad that no one was there to tell me it wasn't real — what's the harm in Dad flashing me that same familiar smile, leaving me warm inside at the memory of it? Let me have my fantasy; it's more than most have. Doesn't anyone who has grieved for a lost loved one tell themselves they'd exchange all of their worldly possessions for just five minutes back in their company? And just like the fog that descends on my day, the only thing we know for sure is what that doctor said, that it will pass. Logic doesn't always have to win the day. Perhaps there is no harm, on some occasions, letting the disease win once in a while.

The pub was closed and you were the only one there, three or four years old, toddling between the tables, everything seeming so large and looming; tables and chairs to crawl over or under, shiny bottles of all different colours neatly stacked behind the bar, windows too tall to see out of even on tippy-toes. Mum and Dad were upstairs keeping the books or taking barrels down to the cellar before the customers arrived. You peered on to the tables, two tiny hands clutching the sides, your toes reaching for the ends of your shoes, the ashtrays overflowing with cigarette ends, too early for the cleaner to come.

You picked up a brush and started pulling it across the wooden floor littered with ash and beer mats, over sticky patches where beer has splashed and seeped into the grain. You brushed and brushed, bristles kicking up the dust, and then you heard it — the sound of metal. A coin shot across the floor. You followed it along the floorboards and finally it came to a half. You bent down, hands on grubby knees, and picked it up — a halfpenny. You put it in your pocket, a promise to yourself to buy sweets, and then you collected your brush and resumed your big-girl task. While Mum and Dad busied themselves getting ready to open up for the day, the pub was your playroom.

I check the internet every day, just in case today is the day, and so many days have gone by like that. Then one day there it is, waiting for me; a semi-detached house in the same village as Gemma. Three bedrooms; not too big, not too small; the perfect price. Better than anything is the beautiful paddock that the large sitting-room window looks out on to, a picture framed with trees that will bring birds and other wildlife almost to my front door. It is everything I have been looking for. I send the details to Gemma and she calls to make an appointment to view, and then a few days later here I am, standing in the house that is to be my new forever home.

It's empty, and I glance around at the blank walls, trying to picture what from my house might hang there, or which chair I could put where. It isn't as easy as it once was to picture a new life; my brain has to work harder, and the images don't flash in my mind as I pass from room to room as they once would have done.

It's different now, and I can't think what goes in which room without it all laid out for me. But there is still that view.

'It's perfect,' I tell Gemma as I look out across the long flat lawn at the back, and I don't recognise the way she looks back at me.

'What about the steps up to the front door – will you manage?' she asks.

She knows the old me would have found the snags, would have looked more closely at the reasons not to buy the house, would have very much been guided by the head, not the heart. But I ignore her, going back to stand in the huge living room, bigger still without curtains to hug the window frames, and I fall in love with the paddock all over again.

'This is the one,' I tell her.

Weeks later, and my house is on the market, an offer made, solicitors talking of a moving date. I know the old me would have been excited by the pace of things, but now it feels dizzying, as if each update that arrives in my inbox holds in equal amounts surprise and excitement. As moving day comes closer, I start packing boxes. I do things the way I always used to, instinct kicking in, trying to work on autopilot. *Cupboard underneath kettle*, I write on a white piece of paper that I tape to the front of the first box that comes out of the kitchen. *Cupboard next to the cooker*, I write on the second.

The following morning, though, I come downstairs and pad into the kitchen in my dressing gown and slippers. I read what's written down on the front of the boxes while I sip at my hot tea. *Cupboard next to the cooker?* I puzzle. I open the cupboard door, it's empty of course, but I've no idea what once lived inside it. Whatever it is, it's in that box, all taped up and waiting to be decanted at the other end. But I try something else that day. Instead of the location, I pull open the box and decide to list every item I have put in there. Only I keep forgetting. The black marker pen hovers over the blank sheet of paper as I close my eyes, wrinkle my nose, try harder and harder to get my brain to recall what I just saw in the box. I open it up again. Of course – kitchen utensils. I close it back up, seal it with more tape. Then wonder what I'd just told myself to remember. I undo it again, the whole process taking much longer. The next time I go to put things into a box, I stop. First I write: *mixing bowls, small jug, ramekin dishes*, and then I put them inside, a smile to myself as I tape up the box that I've found a way around the problem once again. If only I could take this disease out of my head and put it inside a box, Sellotape it up and lose it between this place and the next.

As the days pass by, sealed cardboard boxes grow around me and mystery thickens overnight. I come down in the morning and wander my house, lost for a while, the boxes and their contents giving nothing away.

Gemma and I make two more visits to the new house, not to measure up for curtains or gaps for furniture, but just to give me a moment to stand once again at that lovely big living-room window, to look across at the paddock and picture my new life.

It will be just like any other move, I tell myself silently as I stand there. But it's already different.

They were one of those typical couples, the ones where the wife takes the lead; she takes his coat from his arms, she folds it over, sits him down, checks on him – once, twice – then goes off to fetch a cup of tea. I see it a lot, wherever I go. I know they're only trying to help, so why does it always look to me as if these husbands – or wives – are so much more advanced in their disease than me, someone who has no one to fetch and carry for me, to finish my sentences, to decide that I can't even manage the small chores that are still very much physically and mentally possible. But there's something else I notice about these couples too. I sit with this man while his wife fetches a cup of tea, and I see the guilt written large across his face, in every pore or fine line that reveals more about the years gone by than his memory can recall. She comes back and sits down with us again.

'We were planning on going to see our son in America,' she says. 'But of course, we can't do that now.' I don't know this woman, but the sting in her tone is unmissable. 'Nor see those dear little grandchildren of ours,' she adds.

Her husband sits beside her. He's staring into his lap now. Those lines made deeper with the weight of the guilt.

'You could go on your own?' he tries softly.

'And who'd look after you?' she snaps.

He sighs, knowing she's right, that he and this disease that has claimed the inside of his head are the reason for his wife's unhappiness.

I clear my throat, try a lighter tone. 'Do you see them on FaceTime?' I ask.

The husband's face lights up. 'Yes, we see them often on the screen, clever stuff the technology they have these d—'

'Yes, but it's not the same as seeing them in person.' Her comment instantly extinguishes the twinkle in his eyes.

'Yes, but it's better than not seeing them at all. Just think, twenty years ago we wouldn't have been able to dial their number and then see their faces appear.'

'Twenty years ago we would have been able to travel there,' she shrugs as he shrinks into his chair, the knife twisted further into position.

He glances at me and we share a look. There is no need for words — we understand everything that we are not saying. Neither of us has chosen to have dementia; it has happened to us, and we don't even know why. It is a question that plagues those of us living with it every single day. It steals from us memories, and little dignities that will only grow larger as the disease makes its march on our brain. But it inflicts something else on us: a guilt for the people who walk beside us: husbands, wives, children.

I hate my disease, not for what it's stealing from me now, but what it plans to take from my girls, the havoc that it will wreak on them. It rides roughshod over lives, leaving tattered and shattered skeletal remains where a whole person once stood. Most days, like this man, I focus on what I still can do. I'm grateful for small things like FaceTime, which allows me to still see my daughters and saves me the confusion of a telephone call. But there are other days when dementia worms its way into my thoughts and takes hold with flashes of reality that I desperately try most of the time to avoid. It's not possible then to stay positive, when the losses all come rushing to the forefront of every thought crossing my mind that day, and that in itself makes me lose confidence in myself, my mind, my future, my now. That's the moment when I'm suddenly and overwhelmingly reminded that the future is only a vague concept, the only certainty is my decline – one my daughters will watch painfully.

But it's not just what they will witness that lies heavy inside my head. It's all the vignettes they will have painted of their own future lives that will need to be erased: a doting nanna playing with their children on Blackpool beach, a ready and willing babysitter, a strong and capable mum to see them through all the ups and downs of life. I wanted to be here for so much longer for them, physically and emotionally. Instead it is the other way round; it's Gemma I call when the trains are delayed and I can't work out how to get home, it's Sarah who needs to sit down with me and show me how to navigate a website. Everybody accepts that their parents will grow slower, but they don't imagine that as they do, they will forget the face or the name of the child that had loved them their entire life. That is the cruelty of this disease, that is where the guilt is buried deep.

The new scenes I sketch in my mind are too painful to finish. The guilt then is a motivator: it's enough to make me articulate my future wishes a little more clearly, be adamant that I don't want either of them to be my carer, that I'd rather they leave it to a professional. When they were children I popped them in the bath in turn, soaping their shoulders with warm bubbles frothing with love, and I couldn't bear for them to be asked to do the same for me when I'm no longer capable myself. To lessen the guilt, it feels more important than ever to write down my wishes in the power of attorney document, to sit around a table with my daughter and have those awkward conversations too early.

I remember sitting with another husband and wife at a dementia group. When the wife went to get a cup of tea, leaving us alone to chat, the man told me how struggled he at home remembering where everything is.

'I forget the simplest of things – where the knives and forks are, where I've put things. It's so frustrating. It makes me feel stupid,' he said.

'Have you spoken to your wife about this?' I asked.

He shook his head. 'Oh no, I don't want to worry her. She's worried enough without me adding to it.'

I spotted it again then, the guilt carved deep into his face.

'But how will she know how to help you if you don't talk about it?' I said. 'And how can you help her to understand if you don't talk to each other? If you don't, she'll just make up her own stories without knowing what's really going on.'

His face relaxed a little then. 'Oh, I never thought of it like that,' he said, as she appeared back at the table with three cups of tea. 'Maybe I should.'

If people don't talk about how they feel and the problems they're having while they're still able to articulate them, how can they ensure what happens later, once they're past the point of communication?

When I sat down with Gemma and Sarah to discuss my wishes, laying on the homemade afternoon tea to sweeten the mood, I was surprised to hear how different their thoughts were about what I might want. But I was able to tell them. Imagine the sadness and emotional distress this would have caused if we hadn't *talked*. Imagine the upset and disagreement if we hadn't *talked*. Imagine the distance it may have put between them if we hadn't *talked*. Imagine the sadness I would have caused in my death that I couldn't put right, if we hadn't *talked*.

Guilt is hard to live with, but it exists to help us put things right while we still have the chance.

You never liked to make life easy for yourself, did you? Once you got that career bug, the only way for you was up. You always liked a new challenge: perhaps that's what attracted you to a job all the way up in York. Instantly you remember that junior-school trip you'd made from Ferrybridge to York, happy memories that had lasted a lifetime. Suddenly you were back there, picturing yourself as a child walking along the walls of the city and beside the river, a snaking line of giggling classmates, sunny days and ice creams. It was enough to make you apply for the job. A year later, Sarah moved with you from Milton Keynes to York, you rented an apartment by the river and you could walk to work at the hospital in five minutes. It didn't feel like living and working; you loved the city so much it felt more like being constantly on holiday. The hospital was rolling out a new electronic rostering system and you were overseeing it, and when the contract expired after a year, you couldn't bear to leave the north, so you found a new job in Leeds. You moved there, but you left your heart inside the walls of York city, so there was no choice but to move back and commute on the big blue coastline bus each day.

You found a house, which you called your 'forever home', then you fell in love with it and vowed you'd never leave. But that's where dementia found you ...

Is knowing when to concede empowering in itself? Trapped in limbo, between boxes and homes, waiting for the removals men to arrive, I'm not so sure. The excitement that I know I'd have once felt for this new adventure is lost. I'd usually be planning paint colours or gripped by garden design, but I've noticed this time my brain can't hold multiple plans inside my brain; any solid idea turns to mush with the arrival of another, and everything becomes scrambled and unclear. I focus back on the room, the boxes, my watch that tells me the removal men will be here any moment. Gemma is coming to help me today; Sarah has just started a new job, but she promises me that she will come and visit on her first day off. I'm grateful to my girls for the efforts they make to help, but when I close my eyes and see flashes of images, moves I've made before, I know it was never meant to be like this. I was always the one in control, I had always taken charge, and yet now I need someone to tell me what comes next.

Once all my belongings have been loaded into the removals lorry, I turn my key in the lock for the last time, but I can't avoid the emptiness that clicks inside the catch. Will it be different at the other end? Much like the disease itself, it seems impossible to create a clear picture of what life will look like in my new house, and uncertainty about the future clatters around in the Important Box on my lap as Gemma drives me away from York. The removals men are waiting on the path when we arrive, along with the old owners, who are there to hand me the keys. They've mowed the lawn to save me a job. Once everyone has left, we open up Important Box first and pull out my familiar red kettle, two mugs and some tea bags. A taste of home. I stand again in the big window in the living room, and there on the sill is a card addressed to me. It's from the old owners, welcoming me to my new home. I look around at all the boxes stacked high, little knowledge of what is in any of them, and I realise I have no idea how to turn this house into a home.

'Shall we get started?' Gemma says, sipping at the last of her tea.

We wander from room to room, reading on the front of each box what it contains, my memory of every treasure I've ever collected failing me until we rip open each box.

'It's like Christmas,' I tell Gemma as I lift out a lamp I've had since my twenties.

The fear and panic leaves me then, replaced instead by the excitement that I had been searching for as I start piecing together my new forever home, relieved that it was packed up in one of these boxes all the time.

***

'Didn't you have those clothes on when I came the day before yesterday?'

I've opened the door of my new home to Sarah. She steps in as I look down at my outfit; blue walking trousers and bright green shirt. It's then that the confusion of the day before comes back to me. I only seem to have two sets of clothes. I'd washed this outfit yesterday so I had something to put on today. I'd looked around rooms, poked around in a few unpacked boxes, inside the washing machine, but I couldn't work out where any of my clothes were. Had I left them behind in York, I'd wondered. Or at Gemma's house?

'I don't think I can have unpacked everything,' I tell Sarah. 'I can't find any of my clothes.'

'They're in your wardrobe, Mum,' she says gently, leading me upstairs to the bedroom and opening doors on one wall. As soon as she does, the colours come alive beyond them; rails of blouses, piles of trousers neatly folded, jumpers, T-shirts. Why hadn't I seen these fitted wardrobe doors? I'd been in and out of this room dozens of times. I take the handle from Sarah's hand and open and shut the door a few times. I still can't work out why I hadn't realised they were there. I leave the door open as a reminder and go back downstairs.

Over the next few days I walk past the spare bedroom, each time noticing the open door. I wander in and run my hands along my clothes. I take different things from the wardrobe each day, no longer having to wash each outfit as I wear it.

A few days later, I'm in the kitchen making a cup of tea. It's a tiny kitchen, smaller than my old place in York, and there is a door through to it from the hall, another from the living room. But today they are both closed. I turn to get the milk from the fridge and suddenly I feel completely disorientated. I look from one door to the other, utterly confused. Where do they lead? Anxiety starts to rattle inside my chest and for a moment I'm afraid to open each one, not knowing what's beyond it or where it will lead. My breath is short, my heart pounding. I'm lost inside my house. I reach for one of the door handles and tentatively peer round. It's the living room, still, silent. I wander into it, and then back into the kitchen, closing the door behind me. And when I turn around, it's happened again. I open both doors then, walking out into the hall, back into the living room, back through into the kitchen, one continuous loop taken time and time again until my heart settles back down inside. Back in the kitchen, I notice something shiny on the windowsill – a screwdriver. I take it in my hand and start unscrewing each door from its hinges. I stand them up in the hallway and from there I can see right into the kitchen. Back in the kitchen I can see both the hall and the living room, the anxiety replaced by calm.

A day later, I'm in the kitchen again, admiring the gaps where doors had once stood between the rooms, congratulating myself on the idea to remove them, when suddenly my eyes are drawn to silver handles. I pull on one, it opens a cupboard and inside: 'My cans!' I say to myself. Peach slices, rice pudding, baked beans; they're all hiding inside. But it was the same thing that had happened upstairs; just like the fitted wardrobe doors blending into the wall, my eyes hadn't seen these kitchen cupboards either.

I pick up my laptop, scour the internet for an answer on dementia and kitchen design, and read something about see-through cupboards, but it would cost a fortune to replace them all, plus the chaos behind them would look so untidy. I close each cupboard in turn, testing myself on what I can remember inside. It is like one of those game shows, where prizes are covered over and you only win what you can name, and yet, I can't remember a thing as soon as each door is closed again. The handle is the only clue that anything is inside, and I'm surprised all over again to find cups and bowls and glasses and plates neatly stacked inside.

And then I have an idea. I open each cupboard in turn, taking a photograph of the contents, then I go upstairs and print every single photograph off on my printer. I return downstairs with a dozen pieces of paper, a roll of Sellotape, and on each cupboard I stick a photograph of what's inside. I then go upstairs, doing the same for each space behind each wardrobe door. I stand back to admire my work, a view to what's behind this wall of doors – how will I forget I have clothes now?

I'm smiling as I return downstairs and flick the kettle on, dementia outsmarted once more.

But a few days later I notice there is something else. Whenever Sarah or Gemma come over to the house, they nip and use the toilet downstairs.

'I keep forgetting it's there,' I say. To me it's just a closed door, not leading to anywhere. I walk straight past it every time, and it's not like I can keep it open like the wardrobe doors to remind me.

Later that day I'm in Barnitts, my favourite hardware store. It's an Aladdin's cave that sells anything and everything, even two nails if you only need two. I'm strolling round when I notice a rack of adhesive letters. My eyes fall on the Ts, and I have an idea.

'I'll take these two,' I say, fishing enough coins from my purse to pay for the two Ts.

When I get back home I put one on each toilet door; that way I won't forget.

As the weeks wear on in my new house, I start getting more organised, deciding what goes where, what needs to change. Some people who come to the house comment on the fact there aren't any mirrors anywhere, but more and more these days I find them confusing and disorientating. To me, a reflection doesn't signal where the room stops and starts – just like how getting into a lift is now a tentative thing. I'm never sure where the edge is, placing my feet carefully on the floor, unsure whether I might fall off a ledge. But there's another reason I don't have mirrors: I don't want to see the change that's occurring in me. A few weeks ago I watched myself during an interview and it made me sad to see the person I had become. I didn't speak the way I used to speak, I didn't look how I remembered, and I know that as I age it will only get worse. Also, many people living alone with dementia can find it frightening to suddenly spot another face in their house, so I'd rather just get used to not having mirrors around before I get to that stage.

Is it possible that dementia has changed the way my eyes work or, rather, my brain's interpretation of what they see? Even TV screens are confusing to me now. When they're turned off, they are just black, like a hole in the wall, and there have been many times when I've strolled into the living room from the kitchen and just seen a black blank where my TV once was. For a split second I've had to ask myself whether it has been stolen, and just that momentary loss of reality makes my head spin. I've heard of some care homes covering screens with a picture or a cloth when they're switched off; perhaps I should start doing the same.

The new house is disorientating in other ways too, as I can forget that whole rooms exist. I finished setting up the conservatory a couple of weeks ago: a sideboard on one wall, two comfortable chairs looking out over the garden. I'd told myself it would be the perfect place to sit and stare at the world outside with a hot cup of tea in my hand. Yet the other day I realised I hadn't sat in it once; despite putting furniture in it, I was still using it as a walk-through into the garden. I'd been looking out at the birds, but upstairs from one of the bedrooms, gazing over the treetops, rather than on to my new garden, where the birds hopped around, picking and pecking at worms that raised their heads out of the lawn. It wasn't the room that was the problem; it was the routine I'd got into. The routine made me feel safe, the new room didn't, and so I did what I was used to, what felt right, and meanwhile a whole room was going to waste downstairs. I tried sitting in there, but I squirmed uncomfortably in my seat; something didn't feel right. I sighed, giving up, returning back upstairs and settling down, but it bothered me – it was such a lovely room.

I thought of all the people – families longing to do the right thing – who had created a space in their home for somebody with dementia. I thought of groups I'd attended where people with dementia raised that exact point: how disappointed their relative had been about the thought they'd put into making that special place, but how they just felt uncomfortable there and had wandered back to the old, familiar place. Sitting comfortably, yet guiltily, I thought of my own lovely conservatory and felt that same sting of guilt inside, for nobody in particular. I decided I had to find a new activity for the room, something to shift me out of my old routine, and so I decided to make it the room where I sat to listen to radio programmes and podcasts. And here I am with my cup of tea, looking out on the garden as the robins and jenny wrens weave in and out of the clematis and honeysuckle that grow up the fence, shaking pollen down for the bees.

There were many people who showed you the basics of DIY, but nothing taught you as much as the need to be frugal. There simply wasn't enough money to be wasted on workmen. Why employ someone to do a job when you could just learn how to do it yourself? You started off being taught by your mum; she'd always trusted you to paint the low bits underneath the windows, showing you how to watch out for the drips that ran down the wall, making sure even those tiny hands didn't put a spot wrong. You'd gazed, amazed as she'd hung wallpaper, impressed at how swiftly she went from the pasting table to the wall, easing every bubble out from behind the paper until it was perfectly flat.

The next teacher you had was Terry next door. Once the girls' dad had left, Terry was the one who would give you tips for hanging shelves in the living room. He'd offered to do it for you himself, of course, but that wasn't what you wanted; the whole point was you needed to be independent; there was that hardened part of you left that never wanted to rely on anyone again. He only had to show you once: left hand holds the dustpan to collect the grime, right hand pushes the drill into the wall.

'Are you sure you don't want me to help?' Terry asked again.

'Let me try myself first, and then I'll come and get you when I drill through the wires.' A joke — you hoped.

You waited until the girls were in bed and then sat on the floor with a cup of tea and read the instructions for the shelves again. It's now or never, you told yourself. You marked the walls, just as Terry had shown you, plugged the drill in, and then you began. The wall seemed to shake a little, but you held the drill steady. Twenty minutes later there was a knock at the back door.

'Everything OK?'

'Ta-da!' you said, showing him the shelves sitting proudly. 'I didn't even drill through the wires and fuse all the lights!'

After that there was nothing you didn't want to try. Julie's brother Robin taught you everything you needed to know about the car; how to fill the window washer, pump up the tyres, check the oil. Though you could be forgiven for forgetting some things.

'Where did you say they've hidden the dipstick?' you asked again, while everyone giggled back at you as they perched on the garden wall. They laughed at you, but you wouldn't have known back then how full of admiration they were too.

I drain the last of my tea and pick up my rucksack to leave Gemma's. I've been hiding up in her loft room recently, away from the dust and noise in my own house. It hasn't been easy accepting that this is the first house I've moved into where I won't be the one stripping the walls and putting them back together again, that my white shirt and black jogging bottoms, splattered with the paint of homes gone by, are as redundant as me now. I've gone from being someone who did everything to someone who has to rely on strangers, on workmen to do the jobs that I once would have done. Most people would like the chance to put their feet up, but not me.

I'd quizzed the painter before he started: 'You will use dustsheets, won't you?'

He promised he would, but something inside just wasn't sure. So by the time he'd arrived that morning, I'd gone around covering everywhere in plastic sheeting – furniture, beds – just in case.

'It'll take two weeks to do a house of this size,' he said.

I had to bite my lip, knowing that I'd done a whole house like this on my own in under a week. Back then.

I've chosen grey for the walls and a darker shade for the carpets. Back in September, I visited the University of West Scotland and was shown around lots of different rooms that had been laid out in a dementia-friendly way to help train nursing staff to understand colour through the eyes of someone with Alzheimer's. What seemed most important was the colour contrast between objects in a world where dementia can make so many things blur into one, not just memories, but wardrobe doors that become hidden in walls, for example. In these rooms they had red plug sockets to make them stand out from the wall, and I snapped lots of pictures on my iPad, knowing there would come a time when I would need to remember all these useful things that I'd seen. There were examples, too, of what not to do; laying a busy table with matching table cloths, napkins and plates seemed to me an easy way to confuse mealtimes.

A few days later a man comes round to the house to help me choose a carpet. He sits down and pulls various samples from his case. I know once I would have found it easy to systematically eliminate each one, but this time the choice is overwhelming.

'It's hard enough choosing carpet ordinarily,' I tell him. 'And even harder when you have dementia.'

He puts half of the samples back into his bag.

'Do you think that a soft pile would be a problem?' he asks. 'If you have something that leaves footprints, would you ever think they were someone else's footprints, would it confuse you?'

'I'd never even thought of that,' I say. But I'm pleased he's asked.

He spends extra time going over things with me, making sure we've thought of everything, and in the end, he helps me choose a medium-pile dark grey carpet, something that won't leave footprints behind.

The carpet fitters are not so understanding. I have paid them extra to move all the furniture around and put it back exactly in its previous place.

'I have dementia,' I explain. 'That's why you need to put them back where they came from, otherwise they will just not exist for me, and I'll find it confusing if they're in a different place.'

They nod, chewing gum, looking distracted.

'Perhaps you could take photographs on your mobile phones?' I suggest. 'Just to make sure you remember where everything goes.'

There's a pause and they look from one to another. Was that an eye-roll?

'Don't worry, love, we'll remember to put things back.'

I hang around in the kitchen, watching as they work, but when they move into the conservatory, I know I have to leave; my chest feels tight, my hands clammy. I have a bad feeling about this. As I prepare to leave, I notice the television has been moved out from the wall, the wires hanging helplessly from the back. I quickly snap a photograph of them on my phone, just in case they're not plugged back in when I'm home.

Several hours later I return.

'All done,' they say cheerfully, as I close the door behind them.

I wander around my house, pleased with the colour, happy that the last of the workmen have left. I spot the

TV in the corner, the wires flopping loosely from the rear, nothing plugged back in. I grab my phone and sit on the floor, using it as a guide to plug them back in the way they were.

It's a few days later when I wander into the conservatory and find a vase. I pick it up, let the coolness of the shiny glaze roll around in my hands. Where had I seen it before? And then I think of the carpet fitters. What else was out of place? But of course it's impossible now to remember where it once all stood.

I open the microwave and sigh: another bowl of porridge. Who knows how many days it's been in there. I lift it from the plate. Some of the sticky, milky oats have rolled over the top of the bowl, and I have to tear it from its hardened place, a clue perhaps as to how long it has waited for me. I persuade the contents from the bowl, spooning them into the bin, then throw it into the washing-up. Was that yesterday? Today? Two days ago? Had I eaten breakfast that morning? I stare at the Fitbit attached to my wrist as if it might offer up an answer. It stares blankly back.

I know there was a time when I liked cooking, when making a bowl of porridge wasn't something I needed to plan or set alarms for – alarms I then instantly forgot. Then, there weren't bowls discarded in the microwave, the hardened contents clinging to the porcelain. I know it was different once. There was my favourite curry, my signature dish, all cooked from scratch with pinches of this and that, herbs and spices ground together, the smells that filled my kitchen. There was the last summer I had friends over, when I had to barricade myself in the kitchen with chairs to stop myself wandering off and thinking of something else. It had been stressful making it then, coordinating all the different pots and pans, multitasking an impossible feat. Panic replaces any joy that I once got from cooking.

I cut down at first – no more than two pans on at the same time. I could still make myself a meal then. But when the lids were on, how did I know what was underneath? Too often it would end up blackened at the bottom of the pan, the screech of the smoke alarms ringing long after I'd stopped trying to scour it clean. I made friends with the local fire brigade and they came to fit more smoke alarms in my house, but that just made the ringing in my ears louder when I burned something.

I went down to one saucepan. I was sitting in my chair one day, chatting to Sarah on FaceTime, when I wrinkled my nose.

'What's that awful smell?' I said.

'You're not cooking, are you, Mum?'

She must have seen the flicker of recognition on my face before it even reached my brain.

'Take me into the kitchen with you,' she said.

I found it then, one pan left on the hob, the frazzled contents of something now unidentifiable inside. We made a new rule that she wouldn't call again at mealtimes.

I bought a timer after that, a bright yellow one, which would alert me when I'd left some food in a pan. But it didn't really matter what colour it was if I forgot to set it.

It is not just the joy of cooking that's now lost, but eating too. I've always loved food, mushrooms and chillies in particular, and I'd have them with everything. But more often now I buy them and find them dried and curled up in the back of the fridge. Even my taste buds are forgetting my favourite foods. The way I cook, the way I eat, the way I taste is all changing.

The other day I had some mushrooms. They tasted the same, but I wasn't rewarded with that same delight – the signal sent to my brain, the dopamine released back. It was just a taste, like any other. It had lost all meaning to me. Maybe it's not just my brain that is fading away, but memory in other living cells too. The enjoyment has gone out of food now. I eat to survive, but where is the pleasure in that? And should I forget to eat, a flash on my wrist reminds me, so I make a sandwich, or a salad, something that can't send the smoke alarms into a frenzy. Something bland and tasteless. And I eat it before something distracts me and I wander off and find the lettuce browning and curled on the plate the next day.

It was a funny way to introduce yourself to the new neighbours — up there on top of the shed roof. There were a thousand other jobs to do, but it was a nice sunny day in the overgrown jungle that was the back garden, and while the girls played in the long grass, you decided to tackle the shed roof before another down-pour. It must have been the sound of you banging the new felt on with roof tacks that brought the neighbour outside to say hello.

'You OK up there?' came the voice from the immaculate garden next door. You instantly envied their perfect green lawn and glanced back at your own patch of thistles and weeds, which covered the girls' heads.

'I'm fine thanks, just replacing the roofing felt.'

'I can see that. Not often you see a woman up on the roof. Do you want a hand?'

You tried to disguise the sigh that fell from your lips. You couldn't possibly tell your new neighbour what you really thought of his comment.

'Well, you'd better get used to it, because there's an awful lot to do out here!'

He laughed then, until his wife appeared at his side.

'He'd do well to take a look at our shed roof,' she said, nudg-ing him hard. 'I'm sure that needs replacing too.'

She winked at you as her husband found an excuse to head back inside. You carried on tacking the felt on to the roof as the

girls came and went that sunny afternoon. The new house was in a
cul-de-sac and they loved the fact they could ride round and round
on their bikes as they got to know all the neighbours. They were
back again a moment later, hunting for treasure in the long grass.

'There's a table here, Mum,' they called, their voices buried
in the brambles.

'And I've found an old tennis ball,' Gemma said, holding it
up to the sun.

'A skipping rope!' Sarah cried, as they pulled it from the
overgrowth, pretending it was a snake.

Over the next few days you got it all cut back and the garden
appeared, long and narrow. Once the weeds were gone, the fence
was put to shame, so you got on with painting it, one panel at
a time, watched over by your new neighbour, clearly hoping his
wife didn't come up with more ideas about what he'd have to
get on with next.

I'm on my way home from the shops, turning right into
my new lane, my hand on the white handrail beside the
path, glancing over to the paddock where birds sweep
in and out of the trees that shelter them. I make another
right, go up the garden path, reach the front door and dig
in my pocket for the key. But suddenly something doesn't
feel right. I reach out and the door handle isn't where it's
supposed to be. How could this have happened? How
can a door handle move? I step back, uncertain, and look
again. It's on the right. It's never on the right. It's usually

on the left. Another step back from the door, and then the garden catches my eye; shingle where soil should be. I look around then, notice next door's pots and flowers. *My* pots and flowers. Why is my house over there? Why am I here? I look again at the front door and it slowly sinks in. This is not my house. This is not my door. I scurry back down the path with my shopping bag. I stand briefly at the end of the pathway and look back at them: three identical houses, three identical paths. Mine is in the middle, of course it is. But it hadn't been obvious enough. I hurry up my path, my key fitting into the front door.

It happens again a few days later, only this time my neighbour pops his head out of the door as I head up his path.

'Hello Wendy,' he smiles.

'Oh,' I say, stopping still on the pathway. 'I'll be thinking I own the whole street next!'

'Don't worry,' he says.

But I am embarrassed. I do worry. This isn't me, it's the disease, but how can my new neighbours tell us apart?

A week later I'm wandering around York and come across a little craft market. There are bits and bobs, little trinkets of York, things inspired from all the history around us, but one thing in particular catches my eye, a stall full of brightly coloured tiles, each depicting a beautiful scene of York – the Shambles, the Minster – and next to them, some painted with flowers. An idea comes to mind.

'Do you do these with forget-me-nots' I ask

'No, sorry, not much call for them,' the man says.

I look around, there's no one waiting to be served, so I tell him the significance of the forget-me-not, how it's an emblem for those with dementia, and how useful it would be if I could put one up by my front door.

'It would help me find my house,' I tell him.

It's a moment or two before I see what I'm saying sink in. He takes my email address and promises to be in touch.

A few weeks later a parcel arrives for me. It's heavy and the postman places it down gently in my hallway. I open it up, six forget-me-not tiles stare back, a beautiful light blue that matches their petals exactly, set off by deep-green leaves, and a glaze to make them shine. The very same day an email arrives.

Dear Wendy, I was very touched by your story of how you couldn't recognise your house, he writes. *Please accept these tiles from me.*

I glue one to the wall on each side of my front door that very morning, and stand back to admire how they shine from the path – a beacon guiding me home. What a wonderful gift.

Do you remember that one particular Christmas when you were nine? How could you forget? Well isn't that obvious?

It was never about the presents back then; it was just the make-believe about Father Christmas, the magic in the air, waking up and wondering if he'd been. You'd gone to bed on Christmas Eve, excited as always, squeezing your eyes shut in the hope that sleep would come, followed by someone else. If you listened hard enough, you were sure you could hear sleigh bells. It was like that you must have drifted off eventually.

In the morning the house was quiet and still, no one had stirred and the night still hung at the windows behind the curtains, dawn peering through the gaps at you. You crept out of bed and into the living room, checking round the side of the sofa where any presents would usually be waiting. Only that year there was nothing. The little heart beating inside your chest sank into your stomach then. He hadn't been. Tears made their ways to your eyes for a moment before suddenly you saw the note.

Look in the kitchen, *it read.*

It must have been written by him.

You crossed the hall then and as you did, you stopped still on the floor, your heart, momentarily broken, now fixed and banging away at your ribcage as if it might jump out itself with the thrill of it all. Because right there, propped against the table, stood the shiniest blue and yellow bike you'd ever seen.

It's just one week before Christmas and London is extra sparkly – and wet. I've travelled down to the capital for the Alzheimer's Society's Carols by Candlelight concert at St Paul's Church in Knightsbridge with Gemma and Stuart, and we're in a cab making its way across the city. From each window the world outside seems to twinkle back with fairy lights, and shoppers rush from street to street with bags heavy with gifts. The church is packed with people, six to seven hundred, including lots of celebrity guests, I'm told when we arrive, and I feel my fingers grip the speech that I've written especially for the occasion.

The service starts and we sing so many carols that I know well, the words not lost to dementia just yet. As I sing, I'm grateful for the fact that these songs have survived so many Christmases. There is safety to be found in the familiarity of this season, in the traditions that come and go, marking another year.

Finally, it's time for my speech and I go and stand in the pulpit. Gemma looks back at me from the audience.

'I appreciate the love and support of my daughters whatever time of year, but Christmas is very special for families and has taken on a whole new importance since being diagnosed,' I say. 'Christmas just highlights to me how lucky I am and the importance of having loved ones close by. I know not everyone is as lucky as me, so it's especially important at this time of year to think of those who may not be as fortunate as ourselves. A simple "hello and Merry Christmas" may make all the difference to someone in your neighbourhood this festive season.'

Next a group called Singing for the Brain goes up to the altar. Their choir is made up of people living with dementia, some of whom have already been robbed of the power of speech, and yet music brings the ability to communicate back to them. They sing 'Silent Night' together and as they do, I feel goosebumps up and down my arms.

We leave later that evening and head back to Yorkshire on the train the following morning. It's now just a few days before Christmas and the village is also lit up with colourful bulbs strung up on each house and peering back through windows. This evening, villagers are walking through the darkness towards the duck pond to sing carols together. The crowd gathers around an old-fashioned barrel organ; we huddle together from the biting cold, and I look around at my new community, thinking how the move hasn't been so bad in the end. We sing all the old songs, every one bringing back memories of Christmases gone by, memories that I thought were lost for ever: the shiny new bike, a prawn cocktail, a paper hat slipping over my nose.

The singing comes to an end and the children gather at the bottom of the lane, the frosty air alight with their chatter. There's a flash of light then, Santa's silhouette appears and then the man himself. He walks down the lane, waving to all the children and handing out presents. I see the look on every single face as he passes by, and I can feel it too; the magic is all coming back to me now.

The knives and forks were heavier than the ones you had at home, that's how you could tell it was Christmas. Your mum never liked cooking, so you always went out to a restaurant for Christmas dinner. You'd have done anything to stay home and play on your new bike, but your tummy was rumbling, so you told yourself it would still be there when you got back.

Your dad drove the cream-coloured van and you perched on your makeshift seat in the back, giggling as you bumped up and down, everyone in a good mood because it was Christmas Day. When they opened the back door, you came tumbling out, just to make everyone laugh.

At the table everyone pulled their crackers and, because you were the youngest, all the grown-ups passed the little trinkets that had fallen out of theirs down the table. You stood them all neatly in a row on the crisp white tablecloth. Your paper hat was far too big for your head and kept slipping down, all the way over your nose, so by the time your prawn cocktail arrived, you had to eat with your nose high in the air, your neck crooked back just to keep yours on like everyone else. You'd watch the waiters and waitresses as they busied themselves around your table, wondering every year why they weren't at home having dinner with their families too. When it was time for turkey, there was so much food on your plate you didn't know where to start, but you always had to leave room for Christmas pudding, sifting through the darkened fruit hoping your slice would be the one that had the sixpence hidden inside. You'd search quickly, sure that your spoon would come across the neat package of brown baking paper that it was wrapped up inside. But then a cheer would go up from the other end of the table as someone else held it aloft, and that year in particular your heart sank behind your napkin — until you remembered the new bike waiting for you at home.

For everyone who celebrates Christmas, it's divided into past, present and future. But for me, the past isn't there and the future is too scary to contemplate. All I am left with at Christmas is the present. I am sitting in the living room at Gemma and Stuart's house while Billy curls around my legs, making a valiant effort to tear his attention away from the Christmas tree and the baubles that swing and sway tantalisingly from it. I catch my reflection in one, and for an instant don't recognise the person who stares back. I know this wouldn't always have been me. I feel unease that I'm sitting in a chair, hearing the clutter and clatter of pots and pans on the other side of the wall. What did Christmas mean for me before? There's a blank where other Christmases once existed.

Instead I focus on what it means now. I know that dementia has changed it, even if I can't pinpoint why. It's a time for people to get together, for large groups to squeeze around a table, many on makeshift chairs begged and borrowed from the same guests who sit on them. But I find those big family meals too much now, the clatter of knives and forks on plates vying for attention with the voices that rise up over them, criss-crossing the table in various levels of volume. I know this is why I politely turn down the invitation to dinner at Stuart's parents each year. I'd love to go, but I know it will become overwhelming and that it won't be the me I know there, just a muted version of myself as I struggle to keep up.

I know I can't move the house around like I once did to fit in a six-foot tree. Furniture moved to different places would be too confusing. Instead Father Christmas squeezes alongside the windowsill with my pottery cat. Everyone just has to budge up a bit now to make room for dementia. I know I can't shop for presents like I used to, that the crowds and people would make me panic. And yet I do remember that it was the very same thing that used to draw me before, the chance to watch people's eyes come alive at an exciting find in the shops, to picture the thrill on the face of the loved one they'd chosen to open it. Now if I want to soak up the festive season I pick my moments more carefully. I can look around the shops, but the best times are early morning, or at school pick-ups, when I won't be jostled between tills and aisles by shoppers desperate to get home. And I know that people get sick of all the films repeated on telly over the festive season, but I love to watch them all over again. It's never too taxing trying to keep up, as there is still something familiar.

Christmas used to be a sociable time, but the me now prefers to seek out quieter moments. Billy and I can often be found upstairs in Gemma's loft room, just sitting quietly, taking a break from the TV or the clattering of pans or the friends and family that drop by. People can be offended if you don't want to join in, but big occasions can feel overwhelming for someone with dementia, so it helps to have time to be able to duck out when we need to, and be a part of things when we want to. One woman with dementia told me at a group once how she loved to make Christmas dinner every year.

'Now I'm not even allowed in the kitchen,' she said.

Her family thought it was simply too dangerous, that they were keeping her safe. After all, who doesn't want to put their feet up on Christmas Day? But they were persuaded that letting her stir something in a saucepan would make her feel less redundant.

'I had a wonderful Christmas,' she told me in January, her eyes twinkling at the memory of it, faded at the edges, but still there.

'Well, you can't burn the house down with a wooden spoon, can you?' I say. 'Although it does mean you won't get a load of strapping firemen coming to save you!'

We both giggled like schoolgirls.

It's worth remembering, before another year is out, that even as our memories fade, it's not to late for new ones to be made.

How many times in our day do we take a moment to stop? We spend our lives hurrying from one place to another, between chores, or people, work and home. We feel guilty for doing nothing. Until we come to a moment in our life when something forces us to stand completely still. For me, it was that roadblock inside my head, the one that suddenly made well-worn paths become blind turns. A simple task like stepping into the shower becomes fraught with uncertainty. Two taps become literally a burning question: which one is cold? I have put red and blue stickers on them now to remind me.

There was something else the other day. I put shampoo on to my hair then rubbed it in with my hands, my fingers wriggling inside the stickiness of it, but something didn't feel right. I'd looked down to my feet, but there was no water rushing down the drain, no suds being washed away. I'd forgotten to turn the water on or wet my hair first. There wasn't shame — there was no one to see — just sadness. How had it come to this? Things I've been doing automatically now require so much thought and concentration, reminders even. We understand when babies take their first steps or learn to feed themselves just how many actions and thought processes it requires. It's the same with dementia, but in reverse. Those messages aren't being sent and received like they used to be. They're slow or they're gone altogether.

My iPad and phone ping throughout the day: *eat food, take tablets*. I have to barricade myself in my kitchen with chairs when I'm making a sandwich or a salad so I won't wander off and forget to eat altogether. I came downstairs the other day and there was no washing-up on my draining board. I realised I must have forgotten to have dinner the night before. I looked in the fridge and found the lonely ready meal for one.

So now I embrace those opportunities to stop, to give myself a break from a world that is becoming increasingly hard work to live in. The fountain in York is always a peaceful place to stop among the hustle and the bustle of shoppers rushing this way and that. I don't know how long I've been sitting here enjoying the sound of the water, the relentless whoosh from the jets, a rhythm that isn't too taxing for my brain. The smell of freshly cut lilies floats towards me from a nearby flower stall; smiles from children trying to convince their busy mothers to stop awhile to look at the display in the Disney Store; tables and chairs outside a café, and a violinist filling the air between them with his music, a hat at his feet pleading to be filled with coins in return. And then two smiling faces approach me.

'Hello,' one of the young women says. 'Do you mind if we sit with you?'

I shuffle up, happy to make space.

'You won't remember us, but we're student nurses,' the other says. 'You came to speak to us with your daughter and we loved your talk. We follow you on Twitter.'

'Oh, that's nice of you to say,' I reply.

They sit for a while and we chat. They tell me about their Christmas holidays and the assignments they're writing, and for a second the memory from a few weeks before comes back of the nursing students who'd shuffled in their seats and told me they hadn't expected someone with dementia to be able to speak as I had.

'Even dementia has to start somewhere,' I had told them as they'd sat up and listened that much harder.

We finish our chat and the girls get on with their day, and I decide to spend a little longer in my quiet moment, back to the whoosh of the jets and the chatter of passers-by, just watching, and waiting. For what, I might have forgotten.

***

Do you remember the teenage years, or is that a period you'd gladly let dementia steal from you? With two girls in the house, you'd be forgiven for that. Your career was taking off by then. You were being handed more and more responsibility, confidently running the diaries for the physios, keeping a tally of whom to tell what in your head, never needing to write it down. You realised then just how special your memory was. The switch from running an office to the house was seamless, using the drive home to picture whether the girls had enough clean school uniforms to see them through the next day or whether you'd need to get home and start washing, or think whether you needed to ferry the girls from here to there. Your brain didn't get tired like mine does; it was active and alert deep into the night. It had to be.

You'd go upstairs, collecting newly laundered clothes on the way, depositing a small pile outside the girls' bedrooms. A door would open and the music would grow louder.

'Hey Mum,' Sarah would say.

You'd follow her into her room, sit on the bed, ask her about her day, remembering all she'd told you the day before about dramas with friends and marks due back on assignments.

'I'm starving, what's for tea?'

You'd head back downstairs to start making it. As you did, you'd hear cupboard doors opening around you, a face staring into the fridge.

'How was your day, Gemma?' you'd ask over your shoulder, taking in the details she told you, always interested.

It amazes me now how you did it, because you didn't have anyone to help you. You were Mum, Dad, taxi, chef, counsellor, gardener and housekeeper, all rolled into one. Not that you minded. You batted away the guilt known by every working single mum for not being there at home time. You told yourself you'd find the time to pay them back when they were older. You had no idea that time was finite then, that there would come a day when your roles would switch so dramatically. Back then you were happy to be everything and *Mum. Now, in my shoes, the latter would be the only role you wanted to get right.*

Dementia can be a lonely world to live in. It brings uncertainty, so that sometimes I don't quite know what the world might be today. I miss feeling needed and necessary, and so I work hard to carve myself out a place. At first I found friends in website forums, people to talk to who knew what I meant, a safe space where I didn't need to explain. Back when I was working, I would spend most of my evenings scrolling down lists of forum topics, trying to find the one that best described what I was feeling. Sometimes I was left shocked at the negativity of what I read, at how little it resembled the reality of my experience. I remember a daughter asking users why her mother refused to go into the room she'd newly decorated for her. The obvious answer – that it was difficult because it was different from what she knew as her own room – didn't appear among any of the replies. Instead other carers had written about how dreadful it was, and that this daughter just had to accept it. *Nothing you do will be right*, someone had unhelpfully told her.

They just didn't get it.

But neither did the medical professionals. Our first port of call was the GP, who told me not to bother taking donepezil, because it didn't help.

'So put yourself in my shoes,' I'd said. 'You've been diagnosed with dementia and donepezil is the only medication on the market. Would you discontinue using it?'

He didn't answer. I changed GPs.

During one of the first conferences I'd been asked to speak at, the person before me spoke of the 'challenging behaviour' of people with dementia. It made me so sad that I quickly took a pen from my bag and rewrote a section of my speech to talk about the challenging behaviour of healthcare professionals, whose ignorant responses distresses us. I did it for the many people with dementia who can't communicate this.

Because people don't get it.

And the more experiences I had like that, the more the sadness swelled inside me. So I put myself forward to take part in more and more research. I agree to help select doctoral candidates for Bradford University. I volunteer to be part of research committees, to speak to 200 student nurses and remind them that people with dementia might not remember the detail of their care, but they would remember how it made them feel: a touch of the hand or smile would mean so much. I take part in market research for banks that want to make their branches and online services more user-friendly for customers with dementia. I even take part in the Prime Minister's Challenge on Dementia 2020, because while the aim of the Challenge is to be the best in the world for care and carer support, and to lead the way in research, not one person with dementia was actually on the original panel.

Even they didn't get it.

The retirement that I'd once planned has been lost to a disease that I hadn't asked for, but I am busier now than ever.

I call this my sudoku. Something that exercises my brain, exposing it to new conversations and people and surroundings, week in and week out. Even plotting a journey to London makes my brain throb with confusion. But I do it.

What's the alternative? Sitting around all day waiting for the decline to come more quickly? To allow this disease to make its march even sooner? Isn't it better to keep the cells in the brain that are working well, working for longer?

And there is another reason I say yes to every invitation to speak or judge or listen: because I don't know when this might be my last chance or when people might stop asking me. Dementia has a way of throwing everything into such sharp focus that the weeks when I don't have anything planned make me feel panicky around the edges. What if I forget?

Because I have. I do.

You stayed in the physio department for five years and you were always happy there, but you knew the place inside out, and couldn't shake the feeling it was time for another challenge. You were never one for an easy life. You read in a newspaper about a new initiative, a phone helpline, NHS Direct, and a call centre that was opening locally. After that you scoured the newspaper each week for job adverts, and there you found it one day: health advisor for the helpline. It was shift work, but the girls were getting older. They were more than capable of managing on their own, but still you felt the need to check with them before sitting down at the kitchen table to write your application letter – you were always a mum first. 'Go for it,' they both told you.

You got the job – of course you did – you were so capable, so different from me. You can probably remember the light flashing on the screen, one of the first calls coming in and your turn to answer.

'NHS Direct, Wendy speaking, how can I help you?'

There was a nervous voice on the other end, a woman searching for words to explain how worried she was about her anorexic teenage daughter, how she needed the number of an eating disorders helpline she could ring for her. You found the number and heard the relief in her voice as you read it out. She was about to hang up, when you asked her another question.

'What about you?'

There was a moment of silence on the other end of the phone. You glanced up at your screen, relieved that there were no other calls waiting; a small and rare chance to make a difference.

'You need to make sure you take care of you as well, remember,' you said, a little hesitancy in your voice, a desire not to offend. 'If you become ill, then how will you help your daughter? There's a support group for parents too – would you like that number?'

You were greeted by silence and it unnerved you for a second. You were new to the job, concerned you'd overstepped the mark, but desperate to help.

'N-No one has ever asked how I am before,' a tiny voice finally replied. You could sense the tears that accompanied it. You sighed inwardly.

'Well, you've never rung us before,' you replied, hoping she could hear your smile from wherever she was in the country.

You put the phone down and looked at the brick of a mobile phone beside you on your desk, something you could ill afford, but that gave you peace of mind that your own teenage girls had a hotline to you should they need anything.

In those early days there wasn't a huge volume of enquiries, and so between the lights flashing on screen, one nurse even brought in a roll of bubble wrap so she could lie down for a nap between calls. You'd laugh with the other call handlers each time *the nurse rolled over in her sleep and another dozen bubbles popped, and at the end of every shift you returned home to your girls, confident that as your head hit the pillow, others were also having a better night's sleep for getting access to services or medical help. You realised then, as you drifted off, that knowledge wasn't just power, it was a comfort.*

I pick up my iPad, open its casing, slide the keyboard into position and then I just stare. It's been a while. I'd been so busy a few weeks ago that I felt I had deserved a break, so for the last three weeks my iPad has been idle and this, today, is my first day back. A long-awaited blog entry to write, some research to do, emails to open. I know I'd sat down with a long list, but my thoughts suddenly feel paralysed. What do I do now?

I look from my desk to the window, the blue sky of the outside world for inspiration, and back to the iPad again. Nothing has come to mind. My hands sit in front of me, idle, ignorant of the task they used to perform. There's a scratchy signal being sent from my brain. *Go on*, it whispers, *open the email*. But my fingers don't obey. They don't know how to. I feel it then, that disconnect. The blank that has become an all-too-familiar visitor to my mind. *I feel it*. In the end, I turn it on. There's an envelope icon. Something tells me to push it. I do. There's a red circle with *78* in the middle. Seventy-eight emails waiting for me. I see the name of a friend – Sue – among them. Safety. I push on her name. Her message appears on the right. But I feel lost in this screen, as if I'm trapped behind the glass, a ghostly reflection just visible back. Is that me? Is this me?

Stay calm, a voice says inside. I take a breath, and another. I feel my shoulders sink against their instinctual fear.

I know I usually do this every day and I should know what to do. I tap the screen, but nothing happens. My eyes scan every inch of it, searching for a clue. All I see is my worst fear staring back at me, along with an image of me. I can type words quicker than I think or speak. I *can* type words quicker than I think and speak. But now I can think of nothing.

The thoughts are out of control then, as panic takes over and fear runs across my mind in so many different directions. Is it over? Is that the end of my typing days? If my blog is gone, how will I save my memory? How can I communicate?

Stay calm. That voice again. I slow down my breathing and the thoughts start to settle. *Make a cup of tea*, a voice says. Everything seems better with a cup of tea. I go into the kitchen and am thankful that the task comes to me automatically.

I start again, at the top right-hand corner of the screen. I press the first icon and a new blank email appears. I press the word cancel, then the next button, an arrow. The word *reply* pops up, I press it. The cursor blinks accusingly. What next? I look down at the keyboard but nothing makes sense. I press random keys, using all fingers: *jsjfjksllkksm-fjkfslk*. My hand hovers over the screen, I press *send*. Sue will understand. I sit and wait. Nothing happens.

I close the screen and make another cup of tea. As I boil the kettle I have one agonising thought: what if I forget how to make a cuppa? A smile suddenly appears on my face as I remember all the events I attend where the first thing people do is make me a cup of tea, knowing that they'll immediately receive one of my infamous brownie points. For a second I forget the screen waiting for me in the other room, distracted again.

I sit staring at the birds, the warm cup between both hands. Then I hear a ping. Enough cuts through the fog to tell me it's the iPad. There's Sue's name again. I press it.

What you up to, Wendy? she's written. *What's with the gobbledegook?*

I want to shout at the screen. 'HELP ME!'

The letters on the keypad look like hieroglyphics. They make no sense.

jjdhsufsh I press send.

I keep the keyboard open, knowing she'll be waiting for a reply. A few moments later, the same sound again.

Is there something wrong?

I can read but I can't write.

jknhafapod

Send.

Backwards and forwards like that we go, it feels like hours.

Copy my letters, look on the keyboard and find the same shapes.

I do as she says. I scan each squiggle on the keyboard, press each in turn. Minutes go by as I find each one.

copymyletterslook . . .

Send.

The same again, comes a reply.

thesameagain . . .

Send.

Another reply.

Do you see the long key at the bottom? That will give you a space.

Do you see . . .

Send.

We go on like this, over and over, until one by one the letters start to take shape in front of me. They make sense again. Of course they do.

Thank you, I type finally. *I'm back.*

I flop back in my chair, and slowly my breath starts to steady itself, my heart too. What if she hadn't known what was happening? What if she hadn't known how to talk me back round? Would it have been lost for ever? I squeeze my eyes shut, telling myself not to think like that, but then the thoughts come thicker, faster. It's impossible to avoid them. I feel tired. I have a headache and want to lie down, but I'm afraid to close my eyes. Will it disappear again?

I know then I can't take time off. If I don't use it, I will lose it. I came so close today. I'm scared of losing the last bit of me, the one behind a screen who can type and think articulately. I'm not ready to let her go. I have become used to looking up in familiar surroundings and not knowing where I am, but this was something else. I was lost inside. Screaming to get out. It was terrifying.

I stare at the television as the credits roll. I've just watched a *Panorama* programme about dementia and so many thoughts race around my head. Camera crews had followed two friends of mine, Chris – who has dementia – and his wife Jayne. I know them from the speaking circuit, although Chris's disease is a little more advanced than mine. He, like me, tries to stay as active as possible, even though it is often exhausting.

It wasn't easy to watch the programme and my first thoughts are for Gemma and Sarah, who I know have watched it in their own homes. But one thing I'm left with as the programme ends is how different life is for someone living alone compared to someone living with their partner when they have dementia. Jayne tries to help Chris continue to be as independent as possible. She still sends him out to the garden to get wood for the fire, for example – even if he goes into the garden and instantly forgets what he went out there for. I've seen many people who have dementia whose partners do everything for them, and that only seems to help the disease progress, in my opinion, because they forget how to do things for themselves. Many people that I speak to describe their husband or wife as their 'back-up brain', someone to remind them of things that they've forgotten, to help them when they get lost in the house, to go and get them back if they wander out of the front door at night. But I don't have that.

There are benefits to being alone with dementia. I don't have to worry about someone moving things around in my house and disorientating me. I also have to implement my own coping strategies and these alone exercise my mind, keeping those circuits firing in my brain, the connections tried and tested; the sudoku I do every morning to kick-start my brain while I have my first cup of tea, solitaire on my iPad, and Scrabble with Sarah and my friend Anna.

I manage to travel and get around because I have to. If I didn't, I would just sit at home and stare out at the garden, my brain melting like an ice cream. I have to deliberately make life difficult for myself, going up and down the East Coast Mainline between home and London, across to Bradford, up to Edinburgh and Durham. Navigating my way through Tube stations and London streets. Thank goodness I was always so organised before this disease; many people I know who were never the most organised people, by their own admission, have struggled to learn this unfamiliar skill. I beat dementia by still being organised.

Each week I print off instructions and emails so I remember what I'm doing or talking about every day. I put them all in a pink folder on my kitchen worktop, with train times and detailed instructions about any changes I need to make and printouts of maps and photographs of the building I need to find. Not only does it keep me from getting lost, but it gives me that sense of familiarity when I get there, because I know what I'm looking for. On trains I set an alarm on my iPad to remind me when I have a suitcase with me, otherwise I'd walk off and leave it. A stay in a hotel for conferences could be quite terrifying, but I overcome that by being organised: leaving the curtains slightly open so I don't wake up in the night thinking I'm in my room at home; putting a Post-it note beside my bed before I go to sleep with a reminder where I am when I wake; sticking another to the door to remind me to take the key card. I try to work out how to turn on new showers, but often give up, because even if I do, I have no idea how to change the temperature.

Life is exhausting in a way it never was before. Even remembering to write things on the calendar is challenging, and twice recently I've had to let people down because I double-booked myself. It's happening more often.

I sit in front of the television. Who would know if I wasn't coping? Yes, I have Gemma and Sarah nearby, but they won't know if I get up in the night and head for the front door, or if I leave my living room and forget which way is upstairs. How many more people are living out there alone with dementia without anyone to notice that life has become more frightening, more difficult, more tiring? We don't have the support of someone to cut up our food when we can no longer coordinate the use of a knife and fork. I only know when to eat because an alarm sounds on my iPad. And yet for every clever way I find to combat dementia, it sometimes feels that I am punished for it.

During the eighteen months since I retired, I have been receiving a Personal Independence Payment from the government. It's not means-tested, but based on the practical effects of a condition on a person's life. Recently I was invited for a reassessment and found my way to the office by plotting my route as normal and using a walking app to direct me. The fundamental flaw in assessing people with dementia is that the assessment expects us to recall things, like exactly what we struggle with on a daily basis. But I couldn't remember, of course I couldn't. A few weeks later I received a letter saying that I was no longer entitled to the payment because I can talk normally, walk normally, prepare a meal and have an adequate memory. All of these things are not true. I must have told them how I do speaking for the Alzheimer's Society, but did I explain that I have to write every one of my speeches out and then read it, because otherwise I will just forget what I'm talking about halfway through? It feels like I've had a financial lifeline taken away from me for simply trying to stay out of full-time state care. I feel as though I'm penalised for trying so desperately to cope.

Another thing dementia is stripping from me is my emotions. So I can't even feel angry, just sad.

You were never one to rant and rave. Your anger was usually expressed silently. You didn't need to shout at the girls if they were arguing; simply crossing the living room and turning off the TV was enough to tell them you were cross. Even as a child you didn't have tantrums, so it probably comes as no surprise that anger — an emotion not that deeply bedded inside you — was the one taken so early. There was just one thing that made your blood boil — that inexplicable anger that started deep down in the pit of your stomach and rose up until your head felt ready to explode — and it was the pain you saw in your girls' faces as they waited for their dad to come and pick them up. Once he left he only had to get it right once a month, but he couldn't even do that. You'd see them, up at the window waiting for the familiar sound of his car, their chins nestled into the back of the sofa, their eyes lighting up and dulling a little more every time the sound of a car engine wasn't his.

'He'll be late,' you'd tell them, in your best neutral voice. 'He always is.'

Swallowing down the anger that threatened to burst from within.

'It's probably busy on the motorway,' Sarah would say, jumping to his defence, turning back to watch the cars while Gemma willed the time to go quicker by picking up a book to read, both ears still on the road.

You'd promise yourself that when he turned up you wouldn't say anything; you knew that all would be forgiven instantly by the girls as they rushed up to him with hugs and kisses and clambered into his car, relieved more than anything else that he was here to get them.

'You're late ... again,' you'd say, the anger making your voice waver. Not that it made any difference.

That's what made you mad then. Now it would just make me sad.

I'm walking along London's busy Euston Road. Traffic whizzes by, the sound muffled by the bright-pink earplugs I'm wearing. I look down at my route on the map I've printed, a finger ticking off each landmark – the British Library, Euston Station, Madame Tussauds – it was worth the 5.30 a.m. start, as everything is going to plan. I walk past Regent's Park and the traffic noise fades into the background. I look up at the huge white mansions standing tall behind handsome gates, each garden showing the first signs of spring: a daffodil raising its head to the sunny morning, a purple crocus sitting happily in the shade.

I'm here today to speak at the Royal College of Obstetricians and Gynaecologists and the sense of spring matches my mood, as I've been asked to speak twice today, opening the afternoon session too, and so inside my rucksack are the two speeches I've written, packed with thoughts that I've crafted especially for the occasion.

I arrive at the gates and spot someone waving to me. They seem vaguely familiar and when we meet they tell me it isn't for the first time, but their name badge – unsurprisingly – means nothing to me. I smile, as I always do, trusting what they say to be true. Inside I'm led up a grand staircase lined with the portraits of eminent physicians and into the conference room, where antic-ipation begins to fill the room.

'I know I need to get you a cup of tea, Wendy,' the assistant says. 'We don't want to be criticised on your blog for not having one ready.'

We laugh and I sit happily with my cup of tea, watch-ing the room. To my left an artist is unpacking an array of pencils all colours of the rainbow to sketch us as we speak, and more and more people filter in, everyone chatting and reading through the programme of the day's events. There will be about 200 people here today, but I never get nervous about public speaking, because people's expectations of someone with dementia tend to be so low that they can't help but be impressed when I start speaking. So when it comes to my turn, I start as I always do.

'Please forgive me for reading this, but if I don't, I will forget what I'm here to talk about, get distracted and start talking about something totally irrelevant, like the way I look in the caricature I've just spotted.'

A ripple of laughter goes round the room and I start.

As my speech continues, I watch the faces in the room. Many are taken aback at how eloquent those of us with dementia can be if we're just given the space to be listened to; puzzled faces relax themselves, learning more and more about what it's like to live with Alzheimer's. When I return to my seat, it is with applause ringing in my ears.

We break for lunch and I meet the person who will be introducing me for the start of the afternoon session. I explain where I'll be sitting, but she seems distracted, so I wander back to my seat, my notes for the afternoon in hand, waiting for my call. When it's time, a silence falls over the room, and I shuffle my speech, ready to take to the stage once more. But it's not my name that is called, but Piers, the man who is speaking after me. He shoots me a look from the next table, as confused as me. I glance back at the programme: did I get it wrong? But it's definitely my name first. Perhaps they've swapped us over.

And so I sit there, half-listening to Piers' talk, but the questions roll around in my brain, and the confusion starts to nibble away. After a while I hear the audience applauding, I sit up in my chair, straighten my thoughts and my notes out in my lap. I'm ready to hear my name, but instead it's the next speaker being called. I get up then and shuffle from the room. I feel empty inside. Not angry but numb. I feel hurt, used. On the way out I see one of the organisers.

'They forgot me,' I say.

'Oh, did they? Never mind, you spoke this morning.'

I stand in front of him, thoughts not coming quickly enough, something else rushing to the fore: an uncontrollable sadness. I leave down the grand staircase, the beauty of it dulled by the disappointment of the day. I walk back along Euston Road, tears blurring the path, the traffic making me jump from the kerb, the urgency with which I left meaning I'd forgotten to put in my earplugs. I don't stop until I get to the station. I just want to be home. I get on to a train. I sit. I'm sad.

Being involved makes dementia bearable. But being forgotten ...

The train pulls out of the station.

Words are often lost now. Images are my way of remembering. If I have a conversation, or meet someone new, I probably won't remember the detail of what we discussed, just the feeling I had when I left them. When we meet again, I'll have that same feeling. It's almost like intuition has taken over from the working, practical brain I once had. Those basic instincts have returned. Do I feel happy and safe here? I sense people's moods too; it's almost like I sense an aura of emotion around them, my brain plugging into the bits it can remember, rather than the overwhelming detail that it won't.

I have to work harder now at being a good friend or a mother. I don't want to give up thinking about others – it just takes a little more organisation. Where before I would have juggled what was going on in their lives alongside my own, remembering in the back of my mind if a friend was going through a hard time, or if Gemma or Sarah had a problem at work, now I have to write it down on a Post-it, or set an alarm on my iPad to ask how they're feeling days later. I scan the last email or WhatsApp conversations for things we discussed the day before, so I can ask Gemma how her night out with friends went, or if Sarah managed to fix her car, or if Billy's paw is better.

Today I got a text from my friend, Julie.

Still waiting for news on my new grandchild, she wrote.

Wonderful! I typed back quickly. I was so excited. *I'm so happy for you.*

Yes, the baby was due last week, but hoping it will arrive in the next few days.

I stared at my phone. The baby was due now. I knew Julie well enough to know she would have mentioned it before – several times – and yet it had felt like hearing it for the first time for me.

It's not just bad news we forget – it's good news too. Too often people think about those of us with dementia forgetting that a loved one has died, of grieving over and over. But the flip side is we can celebrate good news again and again too. Of course, Julie enjoyed another chat about the baby. Perhaps it's not so bad sometimes to live in our moment, whatever that moment brings.

People say to me, 'You haven't changed.' It's probably more to do with what they were expecting, what they had prepared themselves for. When friends come to visit, in those first few moments after I open the door I see the way they look at me. They think I don't know, but their faces show that uncertainty, quickly working out how to gauge the situation and how different I might be from last time. Likewise, I see their shoulders relax, the lightness in their voice return, when they realise they haven't anything to worry about, it's still me inside.

Some friends said recently: 'You haven't changed at all since last year – you look the same.'

Perhaps that's what they think I want to hear. Afterwards I thought that I should have asked: 'Just a few more grey hairs and wrinkles, eh? What should I look like? What did you expect to see?'

What is my response meant to be to this comment? There is so much I could say. I could talk about what I do every single day to stave off the symptoms of my dementia, to outwit a disease I know ultimately will win, buying myself some time. That I tire myself out in a world that is not made for me nowadays, that is confusing unless I'm well prepared each time I step outside my front door. Are they expecting the rapid deterioration that you see in some? I am convinced this is often due to 'writing people off' post-diagnosis.

I have to work so hard for people not to notice these differences, because if they do, I don't want the pity that they hand out alongside those realisations.

Friends don't see what I see: that I can't walk like I used to because dementia has changed my gait, that I'm more prone to falls, that I need a stick. That even on a walk around the village I have to stop to let people coming towards me pass, otherwise I get confused about which direction to walk in. A walk in the Lake District that would have taken two to three hours a few years ago, now takes five. I find it frustrating that I can't zip up and down fells and over rocks like I used to. It's not age that has slowed me down, but dementia that has slowed my brain. I'm slower, I'm wobblier, and I have the bruises all over my arms to prove it, but I roll down my sleeves and I get on with it.

They don't see that the condition of my teeth is deteriorating because I forget to brush them twice a day, that the dentist has come up with tips and tricks to help me, suggesting a laminated brushing chart by the sink to tick off morning and night, an alarm in my iPad to remind me to brush, playing my favourite song so I don't get distracted and wander off before I've brushed them for long enough. They're good ideas, but I feel like a child.

I haven't mentioned to my friends that my brain is no longer able to make a simple decision like it once did, that the other day it took me over a week to work out how to book a train ticket on my iPad, taking in three changes and organising seat reservations. That if I don't book a train ticket in a while, I completely forget the process and wonder how people buy a ticket when they want to travel. I want to give up then, when my brain rings inside with frustration. It would be easier, too. But not if I want to win one day after the next, not if I want to stay one step ahead of this disease. But it claims minor victories every day.

I can't use the telephone any more: the person on the other end – especially if they don't know me – wonders why silences fill the spaces between us, and I find myself giving a random response, just to give them something. I agree to things, knowing that saying yes will bring the conversation to an end. Callers speak too quickly, ask too many questions, and so now, if the phone rings, I just stare at it, too weary for the confusion that will follow if I lift the receiver. I allow the answerphone to speak for me, asking the caller to email me.

The other day Sarah and I went to the garden centre and decided to have a bite to eat while we were there.

The choice of sandwiches was dazzling, all sorts of fillings, and yet I looked down at my tray as I went to pay and realised I had the same as always: tuna. Why is it always tuna? Every single time. Because anything else is too stressful, I know I like tuna and so I choose that, and I tell myself that I am in control, that I am choosing tuna to avoid the stress of having to make another decision. But who am I trying to kid? That's not me in control – it's dementia. It's just seduced me into working with it, not against it.

People have looked at my blog and questioned how I can possibly have dementia. They wonder how someone with a diseased brain can possibly write so fluently. I'm thankful that part of my brain isn't broken, that while words lose themselves on their way out of my mouth, the written ones make it on to the page before it's too late.

It's sad when the things you continue to do make people question whether you have dementia. They're not inside my brain to hear or see the hallucinations. Would it make them feel better to see me on a foggy day, the type where I curl up under my duvet and hide away from the world? Would that make the disease fit better into the pigeonhole they've allocated it? I'm pleased that I have broken the mould by challenging myself while I still have the chance, but how much more difficult does that make my life because those around me don't see this invisible disease?

'You haven't changed,' they say. But I used to run and cook and bake and work and drive. I survive now by adapting, by focusing on what I can do. But I don't recognise me, the person who was so fiercely independent and yet now has to accept help. I do what I can. I potter in my daughters' gardens because it makes me feel useful; I watch seeds flourish and thrive and it makes me feel happy. I enjoy eating the food that they make for me because I can no longer cook for myself. I limit my time with my friends to two hours because anything else will leave me foggy and unable to concentrate, but this way, at least, I can still see them.

But there are other times when the difference between the old me and the new me hits me so hard it leaves me without breath.

I'm using WhatsApp with a friend, and our conversation has bounced back and forth for most of the afternoon. We've been chatting and joking, not a second's hesitation, my dementia brain hidden by technology. Ten years ago instant chats wouldn't have been possible.

We haven't finished our chat when the iPad rings: Sarah is trying to FaceTime with me. The red and green words – *decline* or *accept* – appear on the screen. I panic inside. If I answer now, I'll forget to say goodbye to my friend on WhatsApp, and so I wait for the ringtone to stop, and end the other conversation. I call Sarah back, her face appearing as always, bright and sunny.

'Hi Mum, how are you?'

I go to speak, expecting the fluent me who has been zipping instant messages back and forth. Instead, something else happens. A stammer, a hesitation, that search for the right word. When I do say hello, it's with uncertainty. I sound almost childlike.

'H-hello. Good ... th-thanks.'

Who is this? Who am I?

Sarah's tone changes, an unmistakeable difference only a mother would pick up on, and our conversation lasts only a few short minutes. We hang up and the screen goes blank. I see my reflection in the screen, the stranger who now inhabits me. I look back at the WhatsApp conversations, the old Wendy, the one I knew for fifty-eight years. But this one, she is an intruder. I am not used to the two versions of myself crossing paths, but it had felt that, for a split second, they had met one another.

There is a fleeting thought. *Can I go on?*

I extinguish it before it ignites. I know this control I have over my disease is an illusion, a trick I use to get through each day. My friends' kind words are ringing in my ears – *you haven't changed at all* – and yet some days it feels there is little of me left.

There was always that buzz of excitement down at the bus station so early in the morning, egg sandwiches cut in quarters for the journey, a flask of tea, and whispers about what awaited in Blackpool. There was no M62 back then, was there? Just a bus that cut across the countryside, most people going for their annual holidays during factory fortnight shutdown, you and your mum among the crowds. One case beside you, early enough to be at the front of the queue to get a seat right by the driver. From there you'd wait the whole journey just for a first glimpse of the Blackpool Tower; it felt like the whole bus held its breath in anticipation of it cutting through the landscape.

'There it is!' someone at the back would say, but it was too early, you knew it would only be a pylon, too shy to contradict but confident you were right.

Your pockets would be jingling with the pennies you'd saved as spending money and when you arrived at your hotel, you'd split your money into the number of days, dividing it equally so you wouldn't spend it all at once. You were organised even then.

You'd nudge your mum excitedly when that famous spire finally came into view, and once you stepped off the coach into the west-coast sea air, the street would be teeming with tourists. People always seemed so happy in Blackpool – laughter and smiles were all around you there. You'd make your way to your digs for the week, happily walking alongside your mum, trying to guess what might be for dinner, although it was always a salad on the first night, served with white sliced bread and margarine, a favourite of yours, something you never had at home, which made your mouth water at the thought.

Once you'd dropped your suitcase, you'd hop on the tram to theatreland to book tickets to all the shows that week. The trams would mesmerise you, and you'd sit with your nose pressed against the window staring out at the sand and sea, a smile stuck to your face. The theatres were overflowing with famous names of the time: Cilla Black, Cliff Richard, Gerry and the Pacemakers were all regulars, and your mum would be front of the queue to get the best seats so you had a show to go to each evening. You said you'd never forget the night when Cliff Richard looked at you in the front row and told the audience how you'd sat so nicely throughout the whole show. He invited you up on stage to collect a beach ball. I don't suppose you remember that now.

Your mum couldn't walk too much, so she'd sit in the bingo stalls that used to line the front of the promenade and you were allowed to wander off on your own — just for ten minutes before having to return to her side. You'd wander along the colourful arcades, listening to the coins crashing out of slot machines, stopping every now and then to drop a penny into them yourself, but always keeping an eye on your watch. As the week went by, you were allowed out of her sight for longer and you'd run down to the beach and straight up to the sea front, standing on the edge, just out of reach of the surf, thousands of people sitting behind you on the sand. It felt like you were standing on the edge of the world, and it was all yours. You'd race back to your mum, never late, never wanting to break her trust, but you kept your mini adventures to yourself; they were your little secret to keep locked away. Precious memories.

I'm on a train, looking out of the window as the world rushes by. The weather has promised to be kind for the next few days and so I decided to treat myself to a little holiday – a trip back to my childhood favourite, Blackpool. The train is packed with others heading in the same direction, noisy children chattering excitedly about all the things they are going to do with the coins rattling around in their pockets. Every now and then one or the other of them calls: 'Blackpool Tower!' and we all look towards the window, even though it is nothing but a pylon rising from behind a hedge in a field. My eyes are glued to the window too; that same anticipation to wish the journey by, to catch a first glimpse of the Tower myself.

When the train pulls into the station, I head to the same hotel on the quiet North Shore. The manager there knows me and reads my blog, so I'm always well looked after. I love the familiarity of Blackpool, knowing my way around, the streets and tram routes imprinted on what memory remains. I step out of my hotel and turn left or right and I know I can walk as far as my legs will carry me, tiring only to pick up the tram on the way back to my room. The trams go the same route – Star Gate to Fleetwood – every single day, so even if I ever go in the wrong direction, I'll always make my way back.

The trams are people-friendly, no steps to climb, each stop announced by an automated voice and clear big windows to look out of, the conductors patient and friendly, greeting everyone with a smile. One man gets on alone. I know from the way he hesitates – that familiar look in his eyes as he shuffles, how he doesn't seem to know what to do – that he has dementia. The conductor takes him by the arm and jokes: 'Let's get you sat down. If you fell over it would give me a load of paperwork to fill in and I'm no good at that!'

He sits a few rows in front of me, both of us staring out at the view. The landmarks loom large: North Pier, Central and South, the Big One rollercoaster, and of course Blackpool Tower. I get off and spend an hour with a cuppa watching people of all ages and standards dancing happily around the amazing ballroom, grey-haired waltzing partners filling their retirement years exactly the way they had planned.

I walk back along the promenade, eavesdropping on conversations as I go, most of them starting with: 'I remember when …' Blackpool is full of the nostalgia of years gone by, of the factory shutdown weeks that saw the beaches packed with sun-baked bodies, of first donkey rides in the sand and dips in the freezing-cold sea. I feel safe here for that very reason, because these streets are the same I've walked along all my life, memories vying for space in my mind, holidays with my mum and as a mum becoming tangled with all the years they have to share.

Gemma and I came here last year. We love the rides on the Pleasure Beach best of all. We walked along, me with my walking stick, looking in awe at the carriages full of people on the biggest rollercoaster, 235 feet up.

'Let's go on,' I said to Gemma, handing my walking stick to the attendant, both of us chuckling at the shock-horror look on his face, but before he could say anything, I was sitting smiling in my seat. Life doesn't have to be dull and risk-free just because you have dementia.

We strapped ourselves in and were thrown around and around, my stomach lurching one way and the other at 70 mph. It was only the next day, when I couldn't remember why my legs were covered in so many bruises, that I remembered just what fun we'd had. A memory made just a year ago, yet sometimes it feels they're the first to go.

That's why I love Blackpool, with all the ghosts from the past that come to walk down the promenade alongside me. The beaches may no longer be filled with as many buckets and spades as the old days, but those happy times cut through the fog.

A few days later I'm back on the train heading home. I stare out of the window heading across the Pennines; the adults doze while the children swap stories about giant jellyfish found on the beach. Soon the coach is quiet, and if trains could speak, the tales they could tell, of love lost and found, memories made for life, hopes raised and crushed. They zip up and down these lines, all across the UK, holding tight on to all those stories and filling up every day with more and more, never to let go, an endless drive of people's lives.

You returned to Blackpool all those years later, this time as a single mum juggling two suitcases and two girls on a train. The three of you stood on the platform, the girls with goody bags in their hands that you'd made to keep them busy on the journey — colouring books and sweeties. They were all smiles, but you just wanted to get on the train and find a seat together, then you could relax. You'd spend the journey just as you had as a child, chattering about all the things you were going to do: the trams, the sea, the arcades, and then the time would come to concentrate on the horizon, a race to see who would spot the Tower first.

The first tram ride always took you to Pleasure Beach; there were screeches and laughter as you went round and round on the merry-go-rounds, got soaked on the log flumes, but you dried off in time to get a taxi back to the hotel to get changed for the evening.

Each holiday you'd get the tram to Cleveleys, just a few miles away, and tradition had it that every time you had a day out there, the girls got to choose a cuddly toy each. Do you remember the year when Gemma picked out the little bear with goggles and a flying jacket, and Sarah chose the most enormous gorilla?

'How are we going to get that back home?' you said.

267

'He'll sit next to me,' she replied. It was simple in her mind, so there was no reason not to agree.

That train ride home from Blackpool was one you were never meant to forget, Clive the gorilla sharing the four seats around the table, and the girls giggling all the way back beside him.

The smiling face is chattering before me.

'Nice to see you again, Wendy,' it says.

I nod and smile, give them what they want, tell them it's nice to see them too. I answer their questions, they leave happily a few moments later, and then Sarah turns to me.

'Who was that?' she asks.

'I don't know, but they were very nice,' I say.

We both laugh.

'Apparently, I met them at the conference last year.' I shrug, happy to go with the flow as always. This is me now, nodding and smiling, never correcting or questioning. I can't: my memory doesn't back me up. The easy option is always to go along with what they're telling me. It was harder at the beginning. I'd stop and think, wrack a brain that would never come up with the answer, and all the time I did, I'd be missing what they were saying, getting confused, unsure. I felt stupid. Not now. I just give people what they want. I don't let them know I have no recollection of them, as I sense it would be hurtful — even from someone with no memory.

It's surprising how many people don't consider that I may not remember them, but when they do, it's quite refreshing. There was one day at King's Cross station in London, standing out of the way on a busy concourse. Suddenly I picked out a voice in the crowds calling my name. A man was approaching with a beaming face, one that told me he was instantly happy to have spotted me, yet I had no idea who he was. I braced myself for the usual conversation; his assumptions, my pretence. But instead he took my hand.

'You won't remember me, but I'm Joe. We used to work together sometimes in Leeds at the hospital. I know Helen.'

Ah, Helen. My friend. An image of her appeared in my head, a point of reference that instantly put me at ease. It was so nice not having to pretend. We had a lovely chat, he introduced me to his colleague, and then he left, leaving me exactly where he found me.

People are forever starting a sentence with, 'Remember when we did ...'

Sometimes I do. More often I don't. If I say, 'No, I'm afraid I don't ...' they'll spend time going over it, and I'll stand there, none the wiser. So now I just smile and say, 'Did we?'

Unless of course it's Sarah or Gemma, and then I can be myself. 'Nope, I don't remember that whatsoever.' And cue the laughter.

Each day in the village life goes on, whether I remember it or not. The ducks still swim up to the pond's edge, grateful to those who've stopped at the village shop to buy them tiny bags of food. The postman makes his deliveries, knowing which dog sits behind each door, which letterboxes to put his fingers through and which to avoid. And the village bus makes its journey between Beverley and Hull. Mostly – when I'm not leaving home before it's even light to get a train up or down the country – I'm on it every morning at 10 a.m. Lots of us congregate at the bus stop for that first bus, people arriving long before it's due to arrive to catch up on the village gossip, saying good morning, knowing one another's names, picking up from conversations started over hedges the day before. I stand amongst them, listening to the time the village was cut off by a snowdrift. I can't remember now how we got on to the subject, but each of them brings the story to life, how even the snow plough had to be abandoned in the lane where I live.

Enjoying the moment and knowing, just like the blizzard itself, the memory of the conversation will leave me just as fast.

'Morning, Wendy,' the driver says as I step on to the bus. He knows everyone by name, which takes me by surprise, because I can't say I recognise this one. Instead I have to trust his memory instead of my own. After a lifetime of trusting your gut, an instinct that is meant to grow more reliable as you age and have all that experience behind you, it can be hard letting go.

I say hello to the bus driver, calling him by the name the person in front said, relying on them to be right.

After giving up my car, I've had no choice but to take public transport. But it hasn't been easy. The village bus doesn't start until ten and finishes at five, so I often have to rely on taxis out of hours. The firm I use is based at the rail station in Beverley, and in the beginning when the driver arrived late, I used to get very agitated, pacing up and down at my window, unsure whether I was to blame. Had I called and booked it? Had they forgotten or had I? I'd ring up if they were even a minute late. I could often tell by the voice what a nuisance they thought I was. But how were they to know why? I had to put it right: after all, I needed this taxi firm.

A few days later I was shopping in town and I had an idea. I stopped off at Marks & Spencer and came out armed with all kinds of treats and biscuits. I peered through the glass screen of the taxi office and immediately recognised the voice of the lady answering the phone.

'I've brought you all some treats for your tea break,' I said. She looked suspicious, until she saw the biscuits. 'I've come to apologise.'

'Well, you know how to get round us,' she said, taking them. 'But what are you apologising for?'

'I'm Wendy,' I said. 'The one who rings even when you're a minute late.'

'Ah!' she said, the recognition spreading across her whole face.

'I've come to explain why.'

As I sat inside their tiny office, I explained my dementia to her over a cuppa and a few chocolate biscuits. 'I panic, you see,' I explained. 'And then I think I haven't booked the taxi.'

The light went on behind her eyes.

'That's OK,' she said. 'I'll let everyone know; it won't be a problem any more.'

They look after me now, even if my train is late. 'Just come to the office and wait with us,' they tell me if the train home from London gets delayed on the line. They almost always have a car waiting for me.

They are the only people I use the telephone with now. They know instantly that it's me; they're patient and wait for me to say what I need to, repeating it all back to me to put my mind at rest. I'm sure the ready supply of biscuits helps. Who would have thought a packet of custard creams could help me feel so safe?

People often ask me how can I possibly do all the things I do on my own when I have dementia. The answer is, with difficulty. But nothing is impossible even for someone with a brain disease. The journeys I make up and down the country are the ones that seem to impress people the most: how I can get a train all the way from my tiny village and turn up at a meeting in London at a place I've never been before? But so much goes on behind the scenes.

Today I've been invited to Birmingham to set priorities for research. I received the invitation months ago, and as soon as I did, the preparation began. I started by printing. Firstly, a photograph of the hotel where I will be staying; next, a photograph of the venue. I check the route and then print off anywhere that needs to look familiar on the day – perhaps a street I'll be walking down, or a statue I will pass. That way there will be some degree of familiarity when the day comes. Soon there is a whole pile of pictures, and they all go into my pink file, ready for when I need them.

I prepare to leave home in the darkness. I'd booked a taxi a few days before. As the time approaches and I see no car from my living-room window, I pick up the phone. They're not surprised to hear from me, of course, and reassure me that the car is booked and will arrive shortly. The anxiety has already started, though, the clock-watching. I need everything to run to timetable so I make my train. I start working out a plan B, just in case. I factor in time to sit and wait in stations, to collect my thoughts, think of the next step.

I make my train of course, but there is a second and third change I need to make, and the worry is nibbling away inside. I try to stay calm by taking photographs out of the window on my iPad; the sun coming up behind a field of wind turbines. The third train arrives on time, but it is very busy. I need to keep my suitcase beside me, otherwise I'll forget I have one, but there is just no room, so I store it in the luggage rack. I find the window seat that I have booked, but someone is sitting there. I would leave them if I could, but looking out at the views that pass and taking pictures is my way of staying calm on a journey that might otherwise be fraught with fear, and so I have to point out that they're sitting in my seat. Often I am met with tuts and sighs, but today the person is very nice and shuffles over without any fuss. I sit down, feeling happy, and immediately set alarms in my phone to remind me to get off the train when Birmingham approaches, and another to remember to pick up my suitcase.

Everything goes to plan, except as we're nearing Birmingham, I hear music coming from somewhere and begin to jig away to the tune, as it sounds familiar, and then I realise it's coming from me — the alarm I set to remind me to get off with my suitcase.

I've arrived. I feel that little bubble of pride, but then I remember: Birmingham New Street, my least favourite station, with all those exits, all those people. I wander around for a while, trying to keep my fears firmly in their box. Many trains have been cancelled and journeys disrupted, so impatient people mill around, fraught workers hassled from all directions, and in the midst of this, I need to work out how to get out of the station. I pull my suitcase over to the wall, feel the coolness of the brick sink into my back as I wait for the chaos to die down. As more trains pull out of the station, I wait for my thoughts to pull in. After a while, I spot a smiley face, I ask: 'Which way out is best?' They show me.

I'm in the street now. It's busier than the station and the surroundings are unfamiliar. I pull the picture file from my rucksack and flick through the printouts, but I can't find anything recognisable. The panic could start nibbling harder then, taking bigger chunks, feeding on pieces of logical thinking. I pull out my iPad and take pictures, experiencing a settling feeling inside, a distraction from the fear, a few moments of clear, calm thinking reminding me what to do.

I spot a friendly-looking café, a neat red canopy and gingham tablecloths. I head towards it and go inside, ordering a cup of tea. I stare into the beige drink, swirling the milk around with my spoon, the warm scent curling towards me, and then I open the walking app on my iPhone, so I can find my way to my hotel. It's only meant to be five minutes' walk from the station, I remind myself. I look up and ask another customer in the café if they've heard of it. They return my question with a blank stare, an apologetic shake of the head. The app takes a while to load, and even by the time I've finished my tea, it's not working. I ask the staff at the counter. They don't know but hazard a guess, trying to help. I decide to head outside when my app slowly churns into action. It says to turn left, to head towards St Martin's Church, and then it freezes. I see a community policeman, who glances at my Dementia Friends badge as I talk. He knows the hotel, but the app is taking me the wrong way, he says.

'It's not far,' he assures me. 'A ten-minute walk along this road, no turns one way or the other.'

I continue on my way, searching all the while for the building that I'd printed out weeks before, and then suddenly, I spot a sign above the rooftops, the name of the hotel in large letters. My shoulders relax as I head towards it, the smiling faces warm and welcoming as I enter the reception.

I find my room and pull my milk and teabags from my case – there are never enough in hotel rooms. Having a cup of tea, I'm already thinking of the morning, wondering how I'll find my way back from the hotel to the station. It's no good; I'll have to wander back right now so I'll be sure I'll know the way. A few moments later I'm back in reception, taking my phone from my rucksack to make notes as I walk back the way I came. Suddenly a siren startles me as a police car whizzes past, so I pull my pink earplugs from my bag and pop them in. The world dulls around me and I feel calmer now, more able to concentrate. I snap pictures as I go, feeling more settled, as if I know this street now, the shops and offices, colourful doors and windows.

I look up at the sky and the light is beginning to fade. I always like to be back in my hotel room before it gets dark, before my eyes lose their sense of perspective, and everything closes in, black and unfamiliar again. In a shop I buy a sandwich and a drink, and then I head back to the safety of my room, looking down at the rush-hour traffic as I sip another cup of tea at the window.

I can't work out how to switch the lights on, so I make do with a bedside lamp. Managing to get the telly on, I leave one curtain open in case I wake in the night and write myself the name of where I am and what I'm doing here on a Post-it note. Just in case.

I wake/sleep all night, my brain scrappy and unsure in the morning. As I pull my iPad from my bag and check to see if Sarah has made a move in Scrabble, slowly the world clears. Now to figure out how to use the shower in this room. When I turn up for the conference in a couple of hours, appearing fresh and familiar with the place, nobody will know just what it's taken to get me there. I pride myself on that.

Why do I put myself through it? What's the alternative? Not to go anywhere and sit at home deteriorating quickly? I don't think so. That wouldn't be me. Dementia or not.

What makes it all worthwhile – the hassle, the preparation, the travelling, the confusion and fatigue – are the people with dementia who come up to me after a speech or write after reading my blog and say: 'I'm no longer afraid.' Or the daughters who tell me: 'Now I know how I can help my mum better.' One lady wrote to me recently: *When I drive through heavy fog or snow, it's always easier and less frightening when I am following the tail lights of another car in front of me. Thank you, Wendy, for keeping your tail lights on.*

I do it for me, too. Being listened to by professionals helps me feel that I'm making a difference, but not being listened to can feel upsetting, especially when I see that things can't be changed or put into practice because of red tape. I say that speaking at events and meetings is my sudoku, but who doesn't get fed up of playing the same game? Sometimes I feel so overwhelmingly tired that I just want to forget about dementia. When those times come, I do try to give myself a week off, but not too long, because otherwise I'll forget to do all the things that are so hard, and then they'll become harder. That is the thought that clings on through the storm. Fear is our biggest motivator.

I've been writing my blog for two years now. Two years of sharing thoughts, of backing up things to memory. Before dementia, I'd never even read a blog, let alone written one, and yet it's never too late to learn something new, not even for someone with a brain disease. A few months ago, at one of the Minds and Voices sessions, I was taking photos of everyone on my iPad when Rita, another lady with dementia, nudged me.

'Have you really just taken a photo using that?' she said.

'Yes,' I replied, showing her the picture of her smiling face.

'Well I never!' she said. 'I'm sure my grandchildren have one of these; I'll ask them to show me our photos.'

I told her a little more. 'There's this thing called FaceTime and you can talk and see people at the same time'.

'No!' she said. 'How can that be?'

We turned back to the session, but I could see her glancing over her shoulder curiously at the red tablet I held in my hands.

A month later, she was back, full of smiles and making a beeline for me.

'My granddaughter showed me how to look at all our photos, and we did that FaceTime thing and she appeared right in front of me, talking.'

Rita was so proud of herself for learning how to use something new. I know myself how cut off I feel sometimes, not being able to pick up the phone and hear a friendly voice at the other end, but being able to see and speak to my girls makes me feel less excluded.

Twitter was another thing that opened up a whole new world. Colleagues in my old offices used to joke that although I worked in an IT environment, I was clueless about technology, so it's ironic that now I couldn't get through the day without it. At first I saw Twitter as a challenge for my brain, trying to work out how to say what I wanted within 140 characters. I spent forever practising but never having the courage to click on that little blue tweet button; sending my words out into the world seemed a terrifying prospect. Then one evening I was sitting at home with the quietness of the room, the darkness tapping on the window outside and emptiness as my companions. I felt lonely, and then remembered Twitter. I opened up the app and there conversations between people all over the world flitted backwards and forwards in front of me.

I scrolled through endless conversations as an observer, until I came across a hashtag that made me curious: *#whywedoresearch*. I clicked on it and found a whole range of medical professionals, including nurses and researchers, all talking about setting up a new initiative and wanting to find patients who would be willing to promote research on Twitter. Their conversation continued as I tentatively typed out my first tweet: *Could I be your first patient ambassador?* I typed, adding a smiley face for good measure. A second later a reply came: they'd be delighted!

Slowly I joined in more, and was quickly welcomed and accepted. In that one evening I found new friends, people I've met since in real life. I even went to the Houses of Parliament with one to promote research.

Now, whenever I'm feeling the pinch of loneliness, I open Twitter and talk to my virtual friends all around the world. Twitter brings the outside world back in.

I open my front door and try to greet the lady standing on the other side of it with a joke.

'If you've come for my brain now, you're going to have to wait,' I say. 'Because I'm not quite finished with it!'

She laughs as she comes in, and I greet her as I always do, offering a cup of tea, taking her coat and hanging it by the stairs. But there's something lurking beneath my smile, a need to make light of things, to avoid – even for a moment – the gravity of the real reason she's here, because we're talking about what will happen to my brain after I die, as I have decided to leave it to medical research.

There is a strange limbo between life and death when you're living with a progressive illness, that balance of knowing that things need to be dealt with, an acknowledgement of the future, and yet this great urge to live in the moment, to think about the now and forget this is even happening. But the nature of dementia means I can't forget: this disease follows me everywhere, bleeds into every moment. As much as I try to adapt to the person that it has made me, there is not a day that goes past when I don't wish it would desert me as fast as it arrived. I want to have conversations that don't even include its name, to be anonymous in the world again.

We sit down in my conservatory, going over the same memory tests we do each time, the woman making notes in a file that will be pored over after my death. I try to shake that thought away, to remind myself why I have agreed to donate my brain to research, to remember how wonderful it would be if, after I'm gone, my brain gives up the smallest secret about this disease, or confirms some scientific thinking. It's a funny feeling, but a comforting one.

She leaves after an hour and I'm alone again in my thoughts. I feel sad and I'm not sure why. We spent the last hour discussing the end, something that I can't face talking about with the two people I love the most, Gemma and Sarah. It makes sense as a mother, of course it does, but these are important conversations to have, and there are others to add to the list, but sometimes I wonder: haven't we already been brave enough?

I know I didn't perform as well in those memory tests as I had before – I looked over her shoulder as she wrote down the results – and felt my heart sink a little further into my slippers. I'm sure that I wasn't as articulate as when she first visited two years ago either, because the spoken word is leaving me. The words are often too hard to find, take too long to come out, and I give up on sentences halfway through, because the point I've been trying to make has deserted me before I've finished forming it. I pick up my phone and look through my WhatsApp conversations, the text that whips back and forth between friends, accompanied by witty emojis that make me and them laugh. But that's the written word. I can't have those same spoken conversations now, and with that thought something flits through my mind: *Can I go on?*

I brush it away quickly; I don't want to think that. I want to turn back to the now, and not have to go down that road, but the now is changing every day. I'm a different me today from the one I was six months ago. A different one then from the one I was a year ago. I'm losing my sense of self, and that is more frightening than anything, because that's all I have — that's all any of us have. The one we call 'me'. Can I rely on this new me, the one with such fuzzy memories of what came before? What about the one who comes six months or a year from now? Will she be able to articulate that she can manage? That she wants to go on?

I reread a blog post recently mentioning a woman at the WOW conference who said she had already booked her place at Dignitas, the euthanasia clinic in Switzerland. I admired her decisiveness and her bravery then, but I know I can't do that — because of my girls.

I'm not ready, either, of course I'm not. But will the me that I will be a year from now know if I'm ready? Can I rely on her to articulate my wishes? I saw a video of me speaking recently, and I didn't recognise the woman who stared back from the screen. I don't know that voice or the way she speaks, so the me I knew for fifty-eight years has already departed. I keep her alive where I can – in a funny blog post, or a WhatsApp message, an email or a quip written into one of my speeches. Is that the real me trapped inside – or is it the one who speaks on the outside? Is one of them a fraud?

I spend my life now reminding people with dementia – or those who care for them – that they can live well. But some, like that lady at the WOW conference, choose to die well too. I would have more choice if I had cancer – at least then I could simply refuse treatment – but with this disease any suffering will go on as long as my brain dictates. I am powerless. Powerless to live the way I want to, and so I scrape back control whenever I can, but many days it feels that I am fighting a losing battle – and I am. But I'm powerless to die, too. I would go to Switzerland if I didn't have to die knowing that my daughters would have to make that return journey on their own. If assisted suicide was legal in this country, and I knew my girls would not be in trouble afterwards if I needed their help, then I would be first in line. The only thing that remains is the question of when, and that is the state of limbo I live in. Do I want to continue long enough to see myself move closer and closer towards the edge of the cliff? When do I say that I'm close enough? When I know for sure – when I'm close enough to look over and see a blank below – will it be too late to say it then?

There are, of course, changes that can be made in between. I know there is an expiration date on how long I can live independently at home. There may be other options I haven't found yet or delved into. How much time can I borrow from dementia by setting alarms in my iPad to eat and take my tablets? These help me continue the basics of caring for myself. The me now doesn't want to go into a care home. But what about the me that I'll become? How will she feel about a care home? I don't yet know her, I've forgotten who came before, and I can't fully trust this me, either. That's why I prefer the now.

Do you remember that race to hospital? You can't have forgotten, not that of all things. You sat there in the front of the car, holding on tight to your swollen belly, the little life inside nicknamed 'twig' for the last nine months, though you had a better name packed away in your overnight bag. You willed the traffic out of the way: it was the only thing you could do, because they weren't your hands clutching the steering wheel, they were his.

A few hours later you were sitting on the edge of your bed, your chin in your hands, staring mesmerised at the tiny being wrapped in pink beside you, swaddled so tight only her tiny, perfect face was visible. You wanted to unwrap her like a Christmas present, to hold her miniature hands in yours, and yet a second later it was enough just to watch her sleep again, glancing every now and then at the little pink-edged card on the end of the cot — more than anything to make it more real to yourself. Sarah Mitchell had come into the world four days after your dad's birthday.

The second time was three years later, and you were still a month off term, but the doctors weren't happy and sent you to a different hospital for another scan. You drove yourself there, never expecting a problem, but two hours later you held another baby in your arms, amazed at all that extra love you found for this one too. This time the little pink card on the end of the cot read: Emma Mitchell. But something about that name didn't feel right. The next day, you heard tiny footsteps coming up the stairs to the ward.

'Mummy! Mummy!' A little voice eager to see what was inside your tummy.

'Look who's come to meet you,' you said, introducing these new sisters.

From a tiny gasp a smile grew.

'When are you coming home, Mummy?'

'Very soon.'

And then you took the card from the end of the cot, showed their dad how you'd written a 'G' in front of it in biro. 'Don't you think Gemma suits her better?' you said.

You promised each of your babies you'd always be there for them.

***

I know there was once another me for my daughters to call any time of day or night when they were stuck or needed a lift home. I know I always went to their rescue. But now there's this new me. Stuck at Leeds railway station, my train delayed and panic filling my belly, I message Gemma on WhatsApp: *The train's delayed*. With a rolling-eye emoji. It's easy to sound calm in writing. But inside my heart is starting to pound. I keep checking the information board. It simply reads: *delayed*. I text Gemma again, asking if she can pick me up an hour later than we'd planned. More eye-rolling. And then the board goes blank. I brace myself for news, but it flashes up a moment later: *delayed*.

I FaceTime Gemma. 'I don't know what to do!'

She must see my panic. Her voice is calm.

'It's OK,' she says. 'Can you get to Doncaster from Leeds?'

'I don't know.' I look around. The station seems busier than when I last looked. 'Oh wait, yes. The board says Doncaster. It's due soon.'

'OK, go and get that train. Text me when you're on it and text me when you get there.'

I end the call, following her instructions when I'm on the train, when I relax into my seat, when I'm on my way home.

She's there waiting for me. My saviour.

It shouldn't be this way round, though, I shouldn't have to be rescued by my girls. When I was first diagnosed we were all in the unknown. Limbo hadn't arrived then, as we didn't know what to expect. Now we live there.

There was the time when I went to visit a hospice and my daughters were expecting me to be home by 6 p.m., but I got chatting. By the time I looked at my phone I had thirteen missed calls from them and umpteen messages. Now they use an app with GPS tracking so they can see if I'm exactly where I'm meant to be. But it just means I get random text messages saying: *What on earth are you doing in Durham?*

A few weeks ago I went shopping with Sarah. We got everything we needed and stacked our bags in the boot. I went to put the trolley back, telling her I'd only be a few moments and somehow got sidetracked with the thought of buying more compost for the garden. By the time I came out of the store, wheeling two more heavy bags, Sarah was terrified.

'I didn't know where you'd gone,' she said, with a worried look I knew so well, the same that would have been plastered on my face had the girls wandered off when they were young.

'I just went to get more compost,' I said.

But Sarah didn't know that, and I'm sorry that she has to worry so much about me. The girls mostly see the best of me, or that's what I like to think. They rarely see me sad, because seeing their faces instantly makes me happy, the love I feel for them covering up any confusion I've had that day, immediately taking away any hurt or emptiness. Perhaps, then, it comes as more of a shock to them when things go wrong and I suddenly need their help.

It wouldn't do any of us any good to wrap me in cotton wool, though. I didn't do it when they were teenagers, as a parent has to let their child make their own mistakes; it's how they learn what they can and can't do. Perhaps my girls think the same about me. They're just there in the background, waiting for the call.

The images come so clearly sometimes: a flashback to another era, a file taken down from the shelf from so long ago. You never know which it's going to be. This time you're just months old, chubby legs topped with a towelling nappy, tiny digits gripping the bars of the cot, and beyond, the flickering flames of the fire. You close your eyes and feel the warmth of it as if it's only yesterday. Time means nothing; you're a baby again, just for a moment. And then the fog lifts and you're back in the now.

The sun shines through the curtains, a new day peers in from the window. I try to sleep, but it's impossible. Not today, of all days. Instead I get up. I'm on the village bus into town for something to do to fill the time, and I look around the shops, stopping for a cup of tea, knowing anything else in my tummy will just spin around and around like a washing-machine drum. Today Sarah, Gemma and Stuart have paid for me to have my first ever flight in a glider. I look up at the perfect sky above me, knowing that's where I'll be in a couple of hours. I'd been so worried it might be cancelled due to bad weather, but there is not one cloud to break the blue. By the time Gemma and Stuart arrive to collect me, I'm home and standing at the door, coat and bag in hand.

'Are you ready?' Gemma asks, a big smile on her face.

'Yes. I can't wait.'

Sarah meets us at the airfield, me bouncing with excitement, the girls far more nervous. We start by watching a safety video.

'You'll need to watch this to remember how to operate the parachute in the case of an emergency,' the instructor says seriously. I feel the girls' eyes on me. I look back at them with a blank face that agrees we'll keep this to ourselves, that there's no chance I'll remember, and so none of us say a word. I must have done a good enough job at convincing him I've taken it all in, though, because then we're driving round to the airfield where other gliders are taking off around us, towed along the tarmac by a regular plane, the glider pilot releasing the rope once they've reached the right altitude. My stomach does another somersault and I'm grateful that I didn't have breakfast this morning. Suddenly I notice one of the instructors pulling Sarah and Gemma aside, not far enough out of earshot for me to overhear: 'Is your mum capable of this?'

The girls look over to me, and for a second I feel sad. I hate people talking about me rather than to me.

'Why don't you ask Mum?' they suggest. The sadness evaporates instantly.

'Don't worry,' I laugh. 'I'm not going to freak out and grab hold of the controls.'

The mood lightens and everybody laughs.

A few moments later it's my turn. The pilot straps me into the front seat of the glider and climbs into the seat behind me. I look around the small space I'm in; there are a couple of levers and controls.

'You must remember not to touch this lever,' the pilot says. 'And keep your fingers away from the hinge by the window.'

I make a mental note to myself, wishing I'd packed a Post-it note and a pen in my red haversack.

'Remember what you need to do in an emergency?' he asks. 'Just like on the video.'

I nod automatically. 'No problem,' I say, trying to resist the image of me freefalling to the ground from 5,000 feet. *But what a way to go*, I smile to myself.

The aircraft is attached to the front of the glider, and I wave and smile at Sarah, Gemma and Stuart, who are all looking far more nervous than I feel.

'You happy to go?' the pilot says behind me, and then we're off, the plane taxiing towards the runway, the rope pulling taut and us following gently behind.

Then, just like any other flight, we're picking up speed, the world is whizzing by and then slowly I see the ground disappearing beneath us, and we're up in the air, climbing higher, the sound of the aerotow plane's engine in front of us. As we climb, I look out of the window down at the patchwork pattern of the fields below us. I turn back in time to see the rope between us and the plane releasing, our tow flying off into the distance and then there we are left, gliding through the air in almost complete silence, just the soft sound of the wind rushing by and the clouds above me looking almost close enough to touch. I'd expected more noise, but this is so peaceful. I spend my time on terra firma trying to quieten the world down, and yet up here, I find silence.

'You OK?' a voice suddenly says behind me.

'It's wonderful,' I say, mesmerised. I look down at my hands in my lap and see my phone strapped to my wrist. I pick it up and start taking photographs, first a selfie of me, smiling away, and then one with the pilot – looking very serious – in the background.

'Do you fancy circling a bit if we find a bubble of air?' he asks, seeming more relaxed now he can see how much I'm enjoying it.

'Oh yes,' I say, grateful for any extra time we can stay airborne. We go up and up, climbing 300 feet a minute. Below me bright yellow rapeseed fields smile from the ground, small towns look more like model villages, and look; there's a house hidden inside a copse — the world giving up its secrets to us. Then I spot a familiar red-and-cream bus on a long straight road, the same one that I've taken to York so many times. I press my head up against the window; the bus looks so tiny from here, it's as if I could pick it up from the road with my forefinger and thumb. I snap pictures all around, the smile never leaving my face until I feel a slight drop in altitude. I check with the pilot — it's time to head back down to earth. The tiny buildings grow larger and larger as we approach the ground, and then we're there with a surprisingly smooth landing — a simple thud and a little bump. I greet our return to earth with a happy sigh.

A red tractor pulls us along the airfield, towards waving arms: Sarah, Gemma and Stuart, their eyes alight, excited to hear what it was like. Will I remember? Can I recall every wonderful moment? I have my photographs, my bird's-eye view of the world. I promise this is a memory that dementia will never steal from me. Have I said that before?

We celebrate with a cup of tea, and then it's time to leave. What's next? Who knows? All I do know is that I must grab these opportunities with both hands while I can. On my way out, I spot a wing-walking poster …

A good day can turn foggy at the turn of a page. It happened today mid-type. The first I knew was when my head was struggling to keep up with the words in front of me. The haze appeared at first, as if I was driving through patchy mist. Everything slowed right down – time and actions – and my thoughts became more fragmented, like wisps, not fully formed. I know what to do now. I'm prepared for this. I need to lie down, or simply sit still. I make it to the bedroom and climb into bed, pulling the duvet over my head, blocking out the midday sun that shines blindingly through the window. And with that the outside world has gone. The me I'm left with is just a shell. The positive me is somewhere else, and instead a numbness, an emptiness replaces my busy, creative mind. I want sleep to come and take me away, to pour its milky anaesthesia through my brain, washing away the mulch and leaving a sunnier day. I glance at my clock but the numbers make no sense ...

I wake. It's still light. Where have I been? The sun is shining into my room, but the duvet is pulled up to my chin. I'm hot and, I realise, fully clothed. I push the duvet from me and lie there, still. I hear music on the radio, but I don't recognise the song. It's a few more moments before I turn to the clock beside my bed: 15.25. Monday 10 April 2017. How long have I been here? When did the fog come down? There is a man speaking – the DJ from the radio. I try to catch his words as they float around the room like butterflies. I pin one, then another and another. It's Steve Wright. A familiar voice. I'm coming back.

I lie there, allowing my head to sink into the pillow, as the trees on the other side of the window grow more familiar to me. I catch, inch by inch, blue sky between branches, and then birds. Time to move. I shuffle downstairs to the kitchen and empty some porridge into a bowl. I add the milk and flick on the microwave. I unpeel a banana and place it next to the bowl, ready. There is no signal from my stomach to my brain and I'm not hungry, but something tells me that fuel will restart the engine. The microwave hums, the sound blending into the kitchen units.

I see birds outside the kitchen window. I wander out to the garden to fill their feeders, but I shiver. There's a chill in the air that the sun can't warm, and so I head back inside to the kitchen and see a peeled banana on the worktop; it reminds me of the porridge. I open the door to the microwave and find the sides of the bowl dribbling with milky oats. Too much milk or the wrong time set? One of them, for sure. I grab the rolled-up tea towel already waiting on the side and fold it round the bowl. I slice the banana on top and head back upstairs. Back into bed, the sides of the bowl warming my hands through the tea towel. The radio is playing the Beatles' 'All My Loving', a favourite blast from the past. I eat, but I'm not hungry. The tea towel is stuck to the sides of the bowl. How did that happen? It must have spilt in the microwave.

I finish my porridge and put the bowl on my bedside table. Reaching for my iPad, I turn it on. I know the process to restart myself. I open Solitaire and tap the cards one by one, slow at first, missing my chance to move them, and then slowly it comes back to me: red ten needs black nine; two of hearts goes on top of the ace.

I'm back, I think. Almost ...

ACKNOWLEDGEMENTS

First thanks must go to Anna Wharton, without whom this seed of an idea would never have grown. It was such a learning process for both of us, but through all the learning was so much laughter – via emojis – and so many shared emotions. Sometimes people enter your life and you just know they'll be there at your side from that moment on, and Anna is one such person.

To Jon Elek of United Agents, a special thanks for seeing the potential in our book and for supporting us so well. Thanks of course to Alexis Kirschbaum for having the foresight to take on the mantle of publisher, and to all the wonderful staff at Bloomsbury Publishing, including Sarah Ruddick, Emma Bal, Natalie Ramm and Jasmine Horsey.

To the Alzheimer's Society, I want to say thank you for giving me some amazing opportunities; and to many others, too numerous to mention, for asking if I wanted to be included in their work.

I'd like to say a special thank-you to Emily and Damian for setting up Minds and Voices in York – not for monetary gain, but simply because they felt there was a need for people with dementia to meet each another. Without this access to other people with dementia and their love and enthusiasm early on, I might have been in a very different place now.

But most of all, I'd like to thank the two most precious people in my life: my daughters, Sarah and Gemma. Without their support, understanding, laughter, love and willingness to learn with me, I would have been totally lost and very lonely.

Please feel free to read my blog on living with dementia: www.whichmeamitoday.wordpress.com

Or follow me on Twitter: @WendyPMitchell

A NOTE ON THE AUTHOR

WENDY MITCHELL spent twenty years as a non-clinical team leader in the NHS before being diagnosed with young-onset dementia in July 2014 at the age of fifty-eight. Shocked by the lack of awareness about the disease, both in the community and in hospitals, she vowed to spend her time raising awareness about dementia and encouraging others to see that there is life after a diagnosis. She is now an ambassador for the Alzheimer's Society. She has two daughters and lives in Yorkshire.

A NOTE ON THE TYPE

The text of this book is set in Perpetua. This typeface is an adaptation of a style of letter that had been popularised for monumental work in stone by Eric Gill. Large scale drawings by Gill were given to Charles Malin, a Parisian punch-cutter, and his hand-cut punches were the basis for the font issued by Monotype. First used in a private translation called 'The Passion of Perpetua and Felicity', the italic was originally called Felicity.